MAGIC HAIR

MAGIC HAIR

My Experiences
with Lace Wigs

Dana Kathleen McElroy

For Meghann,
the light of my life.

Contents

Preface

One day, in 2003, my friend, Robin, and I were at work, talking about hair. We were always up to date on the latest hair trends. Either she or I would find out something interesting, and we'd update each other on our findings. Of course, Robin would always delegate the research to me. All of my friends know me as the 'researcher'. Anything anyone wanted to know, I'd research it to the death.

Robin's hair was shoulder length and healthy, and my hair was relaxed and snipped short in a pixie cut. That particular day, I told her that I found some information on the internet about lace front wigs. We knew that celebrities wore them, and that they were very expensive. She was intrigued, but a seed was planted in me.

Eventually, through my early research, I found a very colorful website that sold full lace wigs, and even better, it had a layaway program! This delighted us, but our journey ended there, as our minds became distracted with nurturing Shih Tzu puppies, selling legal advice, and other money making schemes. Robin returned to her hairstyles (which were great; I still don't understand why she wanted to hide her hair), and I returned to ritually wrapping my pixie cut and burning the tops of my ears with my dreaded curling iron.

Fast forward to five years later, when I remembered all of our plans for 'fabulous hair'. By this time, I'd been through chin length relaxed hair, naturally curly buzz cuts, stiff beauty supply store wigs, and human hair bonds; disastrous, not a good time, and black glue everywhere. My hair had never been long enough for a sew in weave, which is what I really wanted. In 2008, a new era dawned. After two years of exhaustive research, interesting applications, hilarious moments of mortification, and the acceptance of my own curly coils, here's my story.

Acknowledgements

Meghann Hill – my daughter. Thank you for being you.

Andrew Gibson - the love of my life. Thank you for putting up with the hair, and my ranting and raving.

My immediate family - Muh, Da, Wen, Jeri, David, Cedric, Cary Brandon, Colbi, Jarett, Yahtzee, Nasir, Vicki, and Janelle.

Robin Mathews – who began this journey with me.

Demetria Jackson – for 'dishing with Demi' daily.

P. Butler - my "Thelma".

Susanne – thank you for your friendship.

LuvMyHair631 – for 'adhesive on top of tape = no sliding'.

My vendors - Annette Jones and Rex.

Hair Direct – for being my one stop-shop for my supplies.

Many thanks to the internet forums that I'm a part of:

The BHM Lacefront Forum and The Lace Wig Connection: thanks for the sense of community.

Google (for hosting my blog) and YouTube (for hosting my lace wig tutorials).

Part I:

The Journey Begins

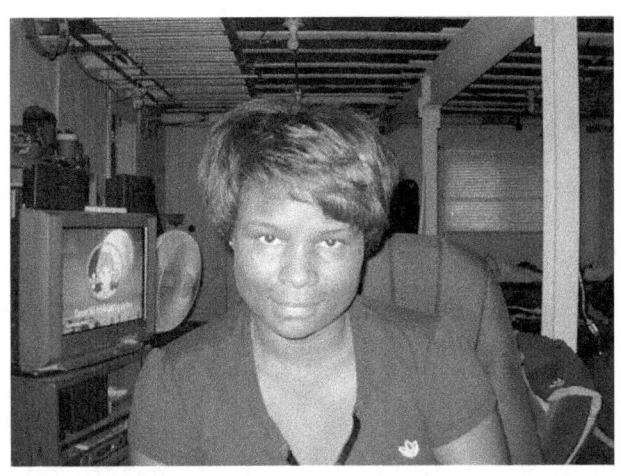

Chapter 1

June 2008 – My "Before"

It dawned on me the other night, that I'm at the point where I think I've done all I can do with lace wigs, other than make them myself. Not that I think I'm an expert or anything; I'm definitely not trying to 'reinvent the wheel'. I'm just at the point that I want to pass on what I know to others that want to know. Yes, I'm spilling my secrets; I'm revealing the mystery. I don't see why what we do with our hair should be kept a secret, especially when it comes to lace wigs. There are so many situations I'd rather not be in, because my lace wig chose to clown, and the people I'm with didn't know I was wearing a wig. The questions I get on a daily basis:

"Who applies your wigs?"

"Do you want to sell any of your wigs?"

"Who's your vendor?"

"How did you get your scalp to look like that?"

"What glue do you use?"

"Can you apply my wig?"

I answer them all as best I can, with all the experience I've gained in the last two years. There are many others that do it better than me and for much longer than me. For the people that find themselves in those situations, and for those who seek my advice on a daily basis, through either my email or my YouTube channel, this book is for you.

This is my testament.

This is how I do it, for all those who ask me. Maybe my tips and tricks can help you. I've been through that dreaded "newbie" stage, of not knowing anything, not knowing where to start, and not knowing where to turn. With a wellspring of patience and a fast internet connection, I was determined to find out all I could about the magic of lace wigs. I didn't think it was fair that celebrities could have "hair today, gone tomorrow". I also didn't want to put up with weave tracks and messy bonding glue. There had to be another way, and I was determined to learn it.

The real journey began in early 2008. All the information I needed was on the internet. I spent hours upon hours searching, and gleaning. There were millions of sellers. So many different wig choices, so many different types of hair, so many different prices. What application methods would I use? Should I get French or Swiss lace? How long would it stay on? Can I get it wet? So many questions. Information overload!

I began bookmarking lace wig websites. I settled on one site that had pages and pages of beautiful wigs. I think the mannequins made the wigs look even better. After looking through hundreds of pages of wigs (with pictures of the customers wearing them), I decided on a long wavy human hair wig. Everyday, I would look at the wig, memorizing the specs and looking at all the color combinations it came in. At one point, I put the wig into the online cart, along with about a thousand dollars worth of adhesives, tapes, mannequin heads, wig pins, and adhesive removers, knowing I wasn't going to purchase any of it. Eventually, the company contacted me, and told me that they couldn't hold items in the cart indefinitely, and that I should only fill the cart if I was ready to make the purchase. I was embarrassed. I let my excitement get the better of me.

Back to researching and being the perfectionist I am, I emailed pictures of the wig I was in love with to my friend Robin. The picture of the customer wearing the wig in an updo convinced us both that we were headed in the right direction. The wig was out of our price range, so it was delegated to the back burner. It still hadn't dawned on me what to do with my own hair.

Finally, after two months of hemming and hawing, researching until my eyes were outside of my head, I ended up ordering a beautiful lace wig from a completely different seller (further referred to as "vendor"). It was expensive, but as a newbie, I didn't know any better. Feeling really shameful, with a wad of money in my purse, I went to the corner grocery store to do an electronic wire transfer. It felt frivolous to spend all that money on a wig, when I was ashamed to wear the beauty supply store wig I already owned (my sister said I looked like the fifth Beatle when I tried it on). With the money transfer successful, the three or four days waiting for delivery seemed like a lifetime. I was more than excited about my new, virtually undetectable hair. One less thing to worry about. I was going to be the first (and only one) on my block to rock fabulous "movie star" hair.

Part of my research was to figure out what types of adhesive and tape I would use. Everything I read pointed to the "sandwich" – adhesive and tape together, so this vendor I purchased my wig from sold all the adhesives I thought I would need: (Oil Resistant White Glue aka ORWG, invisi•bond™ Waterproof Topical Adhesive, Secure™ Silicone Adhesive, Davlyn™ Green Adhesive, and Skin-Shield™ Skin Protect. Supertape™, TDi™ Knot Sealer, and PURE Citru-spice™ Adhesive Residue

Remover completed my order. At this point in my journey, I didn't know anything about body chemistry and if I would be allergic to any of these adhesives. My excitement grabbed me by the hand.

My goodies arrived on a Saturday morning. It felt like Christmas morning. I signed for the box, ran into my room, and laid it on my bed. I stared at it. I was scared to open it. What if I couldn't install it? What if I looked like a fool? What was I thinking? Defeat kicked in before I could get started.

Finally I opened it. It was packed so beautifully, all pink, with tissue paper inside, so nicely folded. There was information inside telling me the name of the wig, the type of hair it was (virgin Malaysian wavy human hair), the length of the wig, how to apply it, how to remove it, and how to wash it. How nice, I thought, how professional. I took it out of its plastic bag and held it up. I was mesmerized. Swiss lace, how delicate. It was so beautiful. I was scared to brush it. I was scared of it. I carefully put it back in its hairnet, then in its plastic bag, then in its tissue paper, and then in its box. I wasn't ready.

Back to the research. For me, there's comfort in research. As long as I'm researching, I'm not doing, which means, I'm not messing anything up. So I began to look up application techniques. How do I cut the lace? How much adhesive should I use? How long does it take for the adhesive to dry? There was no one I could ask for help, because no one I knew wore lace wigs. Through my online research, I found Ms Lola. She is a seller, but she also makes instructional lace wig videos on YouTube. I started watching her videos. She has the most soothing voice, and she likes Jodeci. My favorite Ms Lola video was "How to Keep a Full Lace Wig Bonded Up to 6 Weeks". I watched that video probably over a hundred times, before I ever received my wig. Having Ms Lola's video on was like having her there, instructing me step by step. She used wooden craft sticks to spread her adhesive, which I didn't have. I went to Wal-Mart and bought the economy size package of craft sticks, and a bottle of 91% alcohol (for cleaning up the adhesive). I also purchased a plastic utility cart, with three drawers and wheels, to house all of my lace wig supplies. Back to the project at hand.

At this point, there was nothing else for me to buy. I was procrastinating too much. Truth be told, I was so scared I was going to mess up. I went back home, and had my sister braid my hair. It was so short that she had to add filler (synthetic bulk) hair. It was painful, because my sister braided my hair so tight, but I endured the pain, because I was that much closer to having virtually undetectable hair. I knew I would eventually have to learn how to braid my hair, just in case my sister or my daughter weren't available to help me.

By this time, it was coming up on 5 p.m. Saturday evening, and it was time to get started. No more putting it off. I gathered all my supplies, and sat down in front of my mirror rig (a large hand mirror propped up in front of my computer monitor, and a floor length mirror behind my stool, so I can see the back of my head through the hand mirror, in the floor length mirror). I cleaned my hairline with the 91% alcohol. I put the Ms Lola's video on repeat ("now that's a good bond") and began applying the invisi•bond just outside of my hairline, all the way around my head. I remember that most of the research said to let the adhesive dry until clear. As soon as it was clear, I added a layer of ORWG on top of the invisi•bond. It never seemed to dry, but I forged ahead. I laid a strip of the Supertape onto the adhesives, then a last layer of Davlyn Green. I waited an hour for the layers to dry, and then I applied the wig. It felt so weird.

Here's my very first application, June 9, 2008:

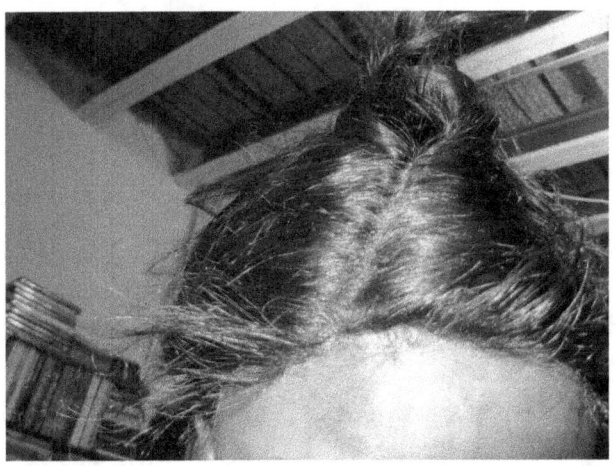

I was so embarrassed about it; I didn't even want to show my face on the photo. I had adhesive everywhere. It took me five hours to do this application. FIVE HOURS. I have no idea why. Back to the drawing board.

I think I used too much adhesive, or the wrong types of adhesive for my skin. It never seemed to dry. I can't remember how long this application lasted. I know it wasn't more than three days. The worse part of my first application was removing the wig. Somewhere along the research line, I realized that I could substitute for products that could be found at my nearest drugstore, instead of always ordering online. I learned that I could clean my wig with 100% pure acetone, readily available at the local beauty supply store. The fumes were crazy intoxicating, and not in a good way.

After prying my wig off my hairline for what seemed like hours, I soaked just the hairline in a bowl of acetone for a couple of hours, until the adhesive floated away from the lace. For the spots of adhesive that didn't budge, I gently brushed them away with an old soft toothbrush. After careful inspection (and totally white fingers from the acetone), I carefully washed the wig with my favorite shampoo. Rinsing thoroughly, then I gently combed conditioner through the hair, and it felt like silk in my hands. After another good rinsing, letting the cool water run down the hair, the hair waved up so pretty. I laid the wig onto a towel and squeezed the water out. I placed the wig on my makeshift hair stand to let air dry. In the meantime, trying to remove the adhesive from around my hairline felt like the devil was doing it. I'm pretty sure I used the whole bottle of the PURE remover during that one sitting. My hairline was torn up. It took a couple of hours to remove all of that gunk from my hairline. I'm pretty sure I lost more than a few baby hairs too. I washed my braids, and put antibiotic ointment around my hairline, and sat under my hair dryer. I was done with my new Sunday ritual. Defeated and exhausted, I went to bed.

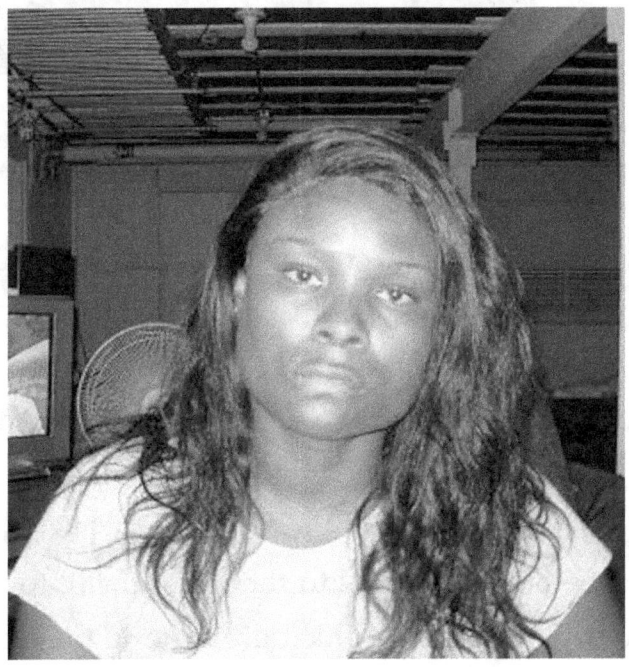

18 inch virgin Malaysian wavy (CLW)

Still using the same adhesives, I tried it again a week later. I can see a white line above my right eyebrow in the picture above. The dreaded glowing 'halo'. Truth be told, I thought I was hot stuff already by this application, but I still believed that everyone was looking at my hairline everywhere I went. Maybe they were, or maybe it was all in my head.

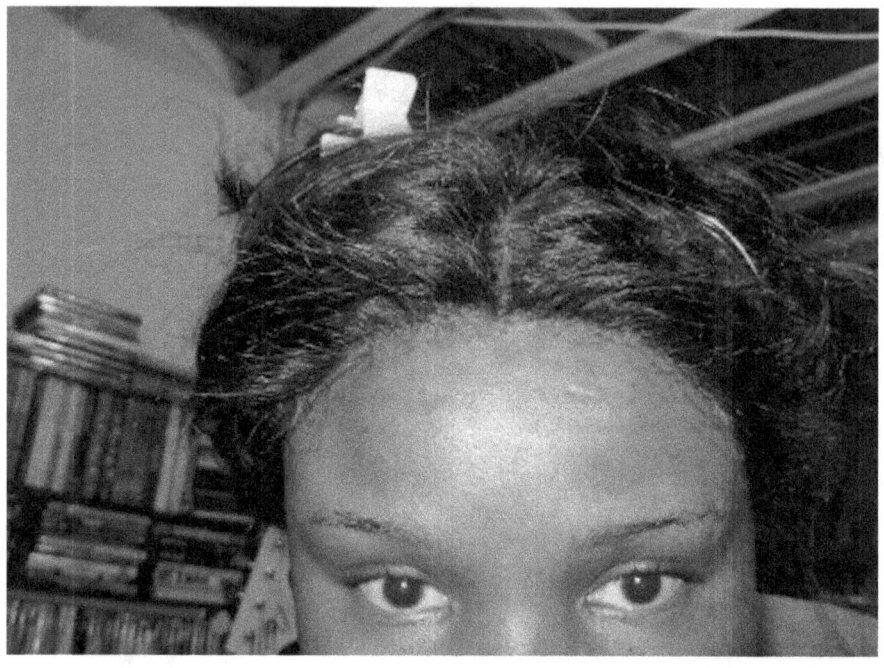

This is what my hairline looked like during the third week. Damn, the white line is still there. What am I doing wrong? I began to rethink the adhesives I have. I added some cocoa brown Rit Dye to the invisi•bond, to make it blend in with my skin. I think it broke down the molecular makeup of the adhesive, because after I added the color, it lost its tackiness. The upside was that my application time was down to two hours. My applications were lasting for three to four days. Back to the drawing board on the adhesives.

Going into the second month of my lace wig journey, I found Hair Direct, an online store to purchase my adhesives and tape. They had everything I needed to apply my wig. I purchased two new adhesives: Vapon NOTAPE® Silicone Bonding Adhesive (from Hair Direct) and Endura-Bond Adhesive (for the life of me, I can't remember where I purchased this from). By this time, I called Robin so she could come see the wonders of the lace wig. I didn't want to call her until I felt like I had the process down (which at this point, I didn't). She came over and she was in awe, even though my hairline was still glowing white. She loved it. She wanted to order a wig immediately. We hung out that whole day, and I felt like people were staring at my head. Maybe it was my imagination. The hair was heavy for me, and I couldn't keep my hands out of it. I wanted to disappear under the hair. I hadn't learned how to "work the hair" yet... a seed was planted in Robin.

The first real test of my new application skills came in August. I was going to visit my boyfriend who lived on the West Coast. By this time, I couldn't get my nape to stick. I'm pretty sure I tore a patch of hair and skin from the back of my neck trying to pull the Endura-Bond soaked lace from it. I turned to another Ms Lola video, one in which she explained how to sew wig clips onto the edge of a frontal. Perfect! I bought some wig clips (from her) and quickly sewed them to the back of my beloved wig. It worked well for me, because I knew how to braid my hair from the nape forward. I left about an inch of hair out, in order to cover the lace edge. I followed Ms. Lola's example to a T. Then it dawned on me – would the metal clips make the metal detectors sound off as I walked through them at the airport? Panic sank in.

Back to the internet in search of anything pertaining to wig clips and airports. Conflicting information all the way around. Just because there was a lot of information on the internet didn't necessarily mean that it was accurate. Well, the clips were sewn in the wig, and the wig was on my head. I did a fresh application the day before I had to leave. I styled the hair in two natural looking ponytails. I arrived at the airport for my departing flight, and I began to freak out. Luckily for me, there weren't a lot of people around, so I went up to the TSA agent who checked IDs. I discreetly told him that I was wearing a wig and that it had clips. I asked him if they would trigger the metal detectors, and he assured me they would not. Whew! Crisis averted. I regained my posture, removed my shoes, put my purse, book, and magazines in the tray, and walked confidently through the scanner. No beeping. No one knew my secret (other than the TSA guy). My confidence level rose up just a bit.

Once I arrived across country, I was cool. No one knew me, for me to be self conscious about whether I was wearing a wig or not. I got my strut on! I had the time of my life. My boyfriend didn't know at the time that I was wearing a wig... until the next day. Everything was going great until I got out of the shower and saw the obvious white halo around my hairline. To top it off, my lace had completely lifted on one side. I thought I could do the 'washing my hair in the shower' thing. I learned in that crisis moment, that the adhesive combination I was using didn't work for water. I was mortified. I locked myself in the bathroom, and frantically searched for my emergency lace wig supplies kit. I'm paraphrasing the following exchange:

"Are you okay baby?" He asked.

"Uh... yeah. Just a beauty emergency. Uh... I'm having a reaction to my hair conditioner." I said through the bathroom door, in a wavering voice. *What to do*, I thought, *what to do?* "I'll be out in a minute." I said, knowing it was going to be much longer than that. A reaction to my hair conditioner! Quick thinking.

I found my emergency lace wig supplies kit. Wooden craft stick, check. Endura-Bond, check. I went to work. After several attempts at laying the lace into the Endura-Bond on my skin, and watching it pop up because my hair was wet, I wanted to cry. Oh Lord, what was I going to do? The only thing I could do. Tell him the truth. I grabbed a towel, wrapped it around my head (no need for him to see the... carnage), and emerged from the bathroom.

"Baby, I've got something to tell you." I said in a somber voice.

"What?" He said, concerned. "What's wrong?"

"I don't know how to say this..." I said, really not knowing how to say this.

"Just say it." I could hear the tension in his voice.

No need to prolong my agony. No way out of this situation. Damn.

"Baby, my hair isn't acting right."

"What do you mean?"

"I... uh... this is a wig. I'm wearing a wig, and the adhesive that I use to apply it isn't working. There, I said it. I'm wearing a wig." I felt so defeated.

"Is that all? I thought you were going to say that you used to be a man or something." He said, laughing. "Why do you wear a wig?"

"Because I'm trying to grow out my hair." I said, relieved.

"Oh, okay. Do what you have to, so we can leave. I want to get the day started."

Right at this moment, I knew it didn't matter to him, and that I got all worked up over nothing. After this scenario happened, I never again felt self conscious with my hair or my wigs when it came to my boyfriend. As much time as I spend on my applications, and researching, there is no way my boyfriend couldn't know what's going on with my hair.

So that's how I'm opening my journey, to explain that I was a newbie, like everyone else who enjoys wearing lace wigs. I've gone through epic and monumental moments of mortification. I've progressed through them to get to this point, where I get asked daily for advice on wig selection, vendor selection, or how to improve an application. This book is for everyone who wants to learn my methods for applying, removing, and maintaining lace wigs. These are the methods that work for me. I didn't necessarily invent them, but I have tweaked them to fit what I need, to have applications that I can be confident in. Hopefully, this book will help answer some of your questions.

Part II:

Lace Wigs 101

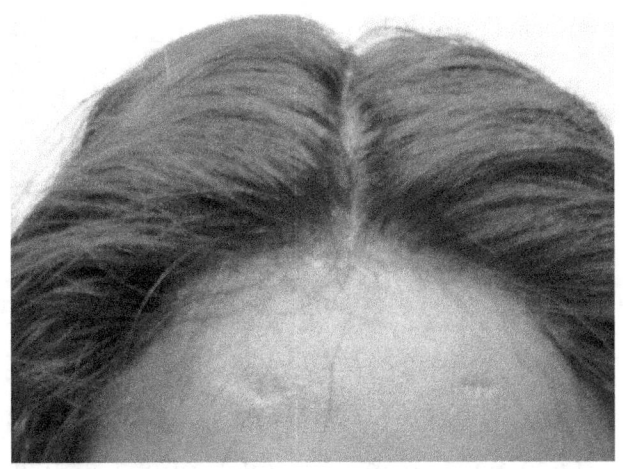
18 inch virgin Malaysian Loose Curly (Rex)

Chapter 2
General Information

The one thing I keep mind when I'm answering someone's question about lace wigs is that I was a newbie. I wore the newbie shoes. I had a million and one questions. I was a newbie on the internet forum (that I still frequent). At the time I joined, I was too scared to jump in. So I lurked. I studied all the posts, I read all the threads, and I read again. I still recommend reading, but a lot of people want a fast track to the best application. They want to skip ahead and attempt an application, become frustrated because the app is whack, and then totally give up. Funny thing is, and I learned the hard way, that although I researched until my eyes popped out of my head, my apps didn't get better until around the fourth or fifth month of doing them. All the links I bookmarked didn't prevent me from having a white hairline the first three months of wearing lace fronts. It's been said a million times, and I'm saying it again. Practice makes perfect.

The hobby of lace wigs (because that's what it becomes, if not a lifestyle) isn't for the person that doesn't like to read, doesn't like to tweak, or doesn't have the patience. Lace wigs aren't for everyone. I still have bad apps from time to time, especially if I'm rushing. I believe that practice and patience are a newbie's two best friends, when it comes to lace wig applications. Since I can't provide either, I'll begin with a little lace wig education. I believe that the skill of applications can be mastered.

This information, in no way, claims to be the definitive guide to all things lace wigs. These are just the methods that work for me.

Lace Wigs

Lace wigs are wigs and hairpieces (toupees) with a lace base. The hair, synthetic, human, or yak, is hand tied to the lace, which is made of nylon. The lace caps can be constructed in various ways, with different types of materials such as stretch lace, silk tops, polyurethane thin skin, or they can be all lace.

Lace wigs are used extensively in theatrical and movie productions, because of their versatility, in color, length, and style. They are very popular with celebrities, as they add glamour and versatility to the celebrity image. Lace wigs are becoming more popular with regular, everyday people, and people with hair loss due to medical conditions, as they are more realistic looking than regular beauty supply store wigs.

High quality synthetic lace wigs are now being offered by various vendors. Vendors can also mimic many hair textures. This option would be a good way to go if you're trying lace wigs for the first time, and you don't want to spend a lot of money. Synthetic lace wigs are applied the same way human hair lace wigs are. I've never had a synthetic lace wig, so I can't give any personal experience on how they behave.

Types of Lace

The two types of lace I'm familiar with are French lace and Swiss lace. French lace is a heavier lace, usually recommended for newbies. It's more durable, but also more noticeable. Swiss lace is thinner than French lace. It's not as noticeable, but to a trained eye, it can still be seen. It also tears easily if pulled (keep this in mind for any activities that would include hair pulling). I try to be as gentle as I can when handling my Swiss lace wigs.

I have to be honest - I purchased Swiss lace for my first wig. I didn't want noticeable lace sitting on the top of my head. Of course, when I started, I didn't know about bleaching knots and simulating a scalp, but I digress. I'm not going to recommend one type of lace over the other. It's about preference. Some people would prefer to work with French lace for their first time trying lace wigs.

The second thing to know about the lace is the color. There are so many different colors to choose, from transparent to dark brown. This is a bit dicey, as there really isn't a way to figure out what color is perfect for your skin tone, other than ordering a wig and laying the lace against your skin. Some vendors sell lace swatches, so that's an option, if you're unsure about what lace color will work for you. Another option is to dye the lace with fabric dye to the color of your liking. The lace is made of fabric, so it absorbs fabric dye. You can also use a fabric dye remover if you make a mistake in dying the lace too dark. Be careful with the dye remover, as it may change the color and texture of the hair that's tied to the lace.

Different vendors offer a variety of different cap constructions: adjustable straps in the back, wig clips in the back, elastic over the ears, elastic in the back, all lace with no stretch material, lace only in the front with wefts in the back, a frontal piece – many different combinations to choose from. When shopping for a wig, I would recommend first looking at the vendor's cap construction section. There, you can see the different caps offered by that particular vendor.

I prefer an all lace cap, with no polyurethane strips (PU) covering the seams. The most common cap offered in stock wigs is the lace cap with the stretch lace in the crown, with PU covering the seams. There was a time when I would only order custom wigs just to get an all lace cap with no PU strips. I discovered that the acetone I was soaking my wigs in melted the PU strips. Since I don't use acetone anymore to soak my wigs in for cleaning, I've begun to use stock wigs again.

Hair Texture and Density

Hair texture in the lace wig world is a point of contention for most. Is it Brazilian? Is it Malaysian? Is it virgin? How much processing has it had? Can you find a true curly Malaysian? What is Yaki? These are all questions that will come up in your quest to find your perfect lace wig. It's all about preference. It's all about what you like. I've gone through a couple different hair textures to find the one I love. I've tried Indian Remy, Virgin Indian Remy, Chinese Virgin Remy, and Virgin Mongolian. I found that Virgin Malaysian hair is my favorite. Since my own hair is completely hidden, what does it matter if my wig hair doesn't match my natural hair? I don't agree that a certain hair texture should match someone's complexion or ethnic group. I'm not that closed minded. I've seen white people with the kinkiest of hair, and dark skinned people with the straightest of hair. What does it matter? Wear the texture that you want to wear.

The process of trying to find your favorite type of hair can be very costly. Remy is supposed to be the highest grade of human hair available for wigs and extensions. All of the hair cuticles are aligned in such a way that the hair isn't supposed to tangle. Virgin Remy is supposed to be completely unprocessed. This type of hair is very expensive. Yaki hair is processed to mimic relaxed African American hair. You can also get processed textures like silky, silky yaki, curly, deep curly, kinky, afro kinky, water wave, deep wave, body wave – the possibilities are endless. Be careful with these textures, when adding extra processing to them (such as bleaching or coloring).

Some people have a variety of hair textures in their lace wig collections. I haven't thought deeper about where my vendor gets the hair from. As long as the hair performs the way I want it to, and as long as it's human, it doesn't matter to me if it's Chinese, Malaysian, Brazilian, or Mongolian. This is an argument that I don't participate in. Just as long as it's not synthetic. I don't like synthetic hair. I like to color and curl hair, and synthetic hair would melt.

Hair density should be noted when considering wearing a lace wig. The density of the wig determines how thick the hair is. Some people opt for a natural looking light to medium density, while other people love densities as thick as lions' manes. Most wig websites should have information regarding the densities of their wigs. Stock wig densities are fixed, but this is a feature you can change when ordering a custom wig.

Hair Length

Again, this is another personal preference. I've had lace wigs as short as 14 inches and as long as 22 inches. I've settled at a comfortable 18 inches. Sometimes I get whimsical and order something different – most recently, a 14 inch virgin Malaysian tight curly wig (already killed, may she rest in peace). It's supposed to be my summer hair... I digress. It's all about preference, mood, and what look you want to convey.

Some people measure the hair from where it's tied to the lace, to the end of the hair. Some people measure the hair from the crown of the hair, to the ends. To me, as long as it's at the promised length or longer, I'm happy. I measure from the top of my head, to the ends of the hair. Again, this is not an argument I want to participate in. Some vendors can be generous with their lengths, but the prices rise according to length. Lace wigs can be fantasy hair, so go ahead with your bad self, and indulge your fantasy!

Hair Color

Guess what? Yes, this is another personal preference. Hair for the lace wigs can come in any color you desire, anywhere from jet black to platinum blonde. Lace wigs are a fun way to try out a new color, if you don't want to dye your own hair. Highlights, streaks, chunks, strands, whatever lurks in your imagination. I tend to stay around the 1B (brown/black) and 2 (dark brown) colors. I've tried as light as a 4 (medium brown) but I didn't like that particular color on me. I like my tight curly wigs colored different shades of brown, with blondish highlights. Go crazy with color if you like.

Silk Tops, Thin Skins, Suction Caps

I'm including these three options in the book even though I don't have any experience with them. People still ask me questions about them, so I'll offer my thoughts.

I think the concept of silk top lace wigs is a good one. A silk top lace wig is a wig that has a piece of layered silk fabric in the crown of the wig, with hair injected through the silk layers, mimicking a scalp. The rest of the cap is made with lace, or whatever cap construction you want (if you're ordering a custom). The silk can be dyed to look like a scalp. I'm scared of silk tops, because of two things: not being able to get a good, realistic scalp color for the silk, and when the lace starts to fray in front of the silk. I hear people raving about the silk tops, and I also hear people complaining about the two things I'm afraid of. I've got a good thing going with my setup, so I'm not jumping on this bandwagon.

Thin skin wigs are lace wigs that are made with polyurethane, either around the perimeter, or as a full cap. The polyurethane can be made to match your skin color. This type of wig would be a great option for people who are completely bald, but would not be recommended for people who live in humid areas, as the wig can trap heat and moisture.

The most expensive wigs available are suction caps, or vacuum base wigs. They are silicone base wigs with human hair injected into the silicone. These types of wigs are custom made for women who experience total hair loss. Not every vendor carries this type of wig.

There are many different types of wigs available. I'm just speaking on a few topics that I've come across in my wig wearing experience.

Hair Styling

This is the fun part. Who doesn't like to play with hair, other than my mother? I have several wigs, based on color and style. In my lace wig arsenal, I have a straight 18 inch, a loose curly/wavy 18 inch, both "Malaysian" textured, and a 20" Virgin Indian wig. The 14 inch curly Malaysian is no longer in rotation, because I cut the bangs too short. I still kept it because I intend on ventilating the front hairline of my future wigs with the curly Malaysian hair. Back on track... the reason why I have different textures is because I don't like to over-process my wigs with heat. I use a steam hairsetter (curlers) on my straight Malaysian and virgin Indian sometimes, but for my wavy Malaysian, I keep it loose or I pull it up into a high ponytail.

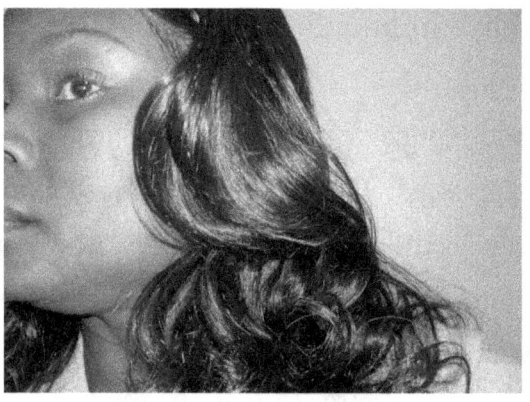

18 inch virgin Malaysian Natural Straight (Rex), styled with ionic steam rollers; layers cut with the CreaClip®

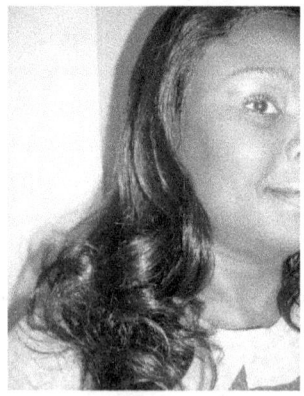

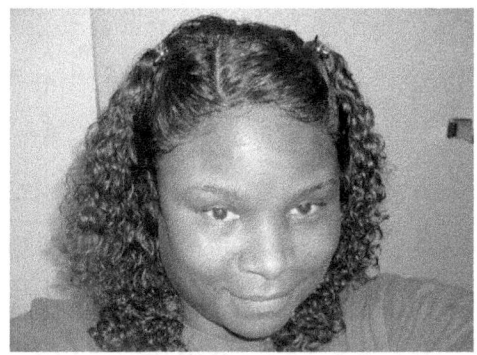

14 inch virgin Malaysian Curly (Rex)

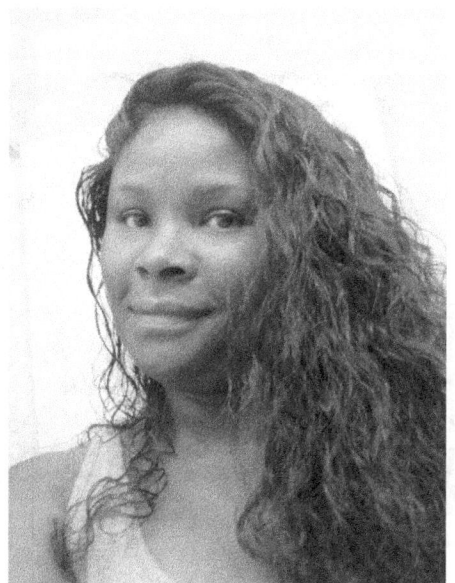

18 inch virgin Malaysian loose curly/wavy

As you can see, I don't do any extra styling to the wigs that are already curled. For cutting basic layers, I use the CreaClip®, invented by Mai Lieu.

I believe that the less manipulation done to the wig, the longer it will last. You don't want to load the hair with product. Mousses and hair serums work better than old fashioned hair grease. I also believe that the key to a natural application is a natural hairstyle. Again, hairstyles are a personal preference. You can be as simple as a part down the middle and the hair tucked behind the ears or as extravagant as Diana Ross, all big and fluffy hair. Don't be afraid to style the hair. This is where your creativity can really shine.

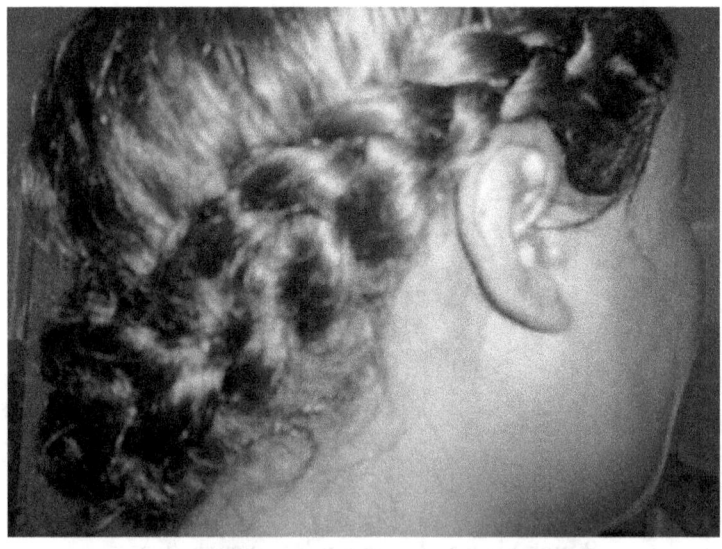

16 inch Indian remy loose curly (Rex)

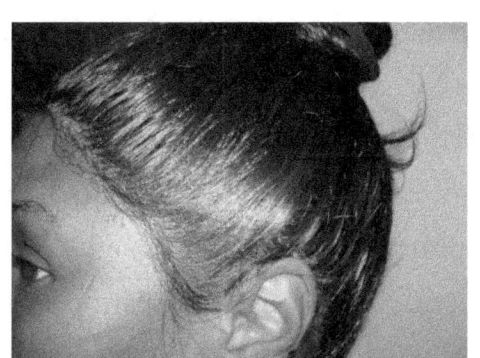

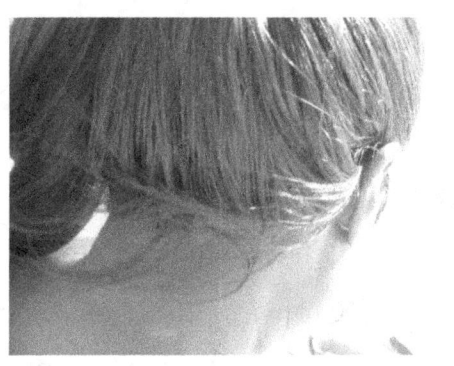

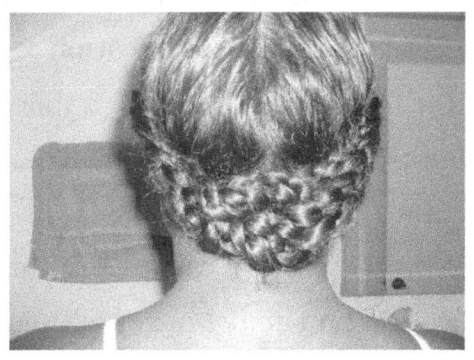

Life Activities

Once you integrate lace wigs into your life, it's easy to carry on your daily activities. I've heard horror stories of how people are at work, and their wig slides back behind their real hairline (or lack there of); or how they're on a date, and their sideburn pops up. Aside from my first moment of mortification I explained earlier, I had a similar moment when my boyfriend and I went on vacation in Mexico. By then, I had found the correct adhesive/tape combination for my body chemistry. My hairline still turned white, after hours of frolicking in the water. I'm the type of woman who's not afraid to get my hair wet. I don't know if that's because I'm a Pisces. I digress. My wig only lifted just a bit in the front (thank God I had a baseball hat with me), but I brought the Endura-Bond with me (always in my emergency kit). This time, I put the hard bond adhesive on top of a piece of Supertape, so the Endura-Bond wasn't in direct contact with my skin. That particular application lasted fourteen days, which is still my longest lasting application to date. However, I don't recommend wearing your lace wig for that length of time.

When we travel, I always make sure I'm prepared to redo my application on site if I have to. I pack Supertape, white adhesive, Vapon NOTAPE, Endura-Bond, enough wooden craft sticks, scissors, cotton swabs, and scarves. I always buy 91% or 99% alcohol wherever we are, just because I don't want it to spill in my luggage. If we fly, I always pack my lace wig application supplies in my checked baggage. I never carry it onto the plane, for fear that they may make me throw it away. So far, I've never had to redo an application while away on vacation.

When I was a newbie, I always wondered if I could swim in a lace wig. From what I've learned, it depends on the type of adhesive, and the amount of layers. If I'm swimming or playing in water, and I know this ahead of time, I consider this a three Vapon NOTAPE layer application (on top of the Supertape and white adhesive). After you're done with your water activities, tie a scarf around your hairline as soon as you can. The adhesive bond tends to loosen up a bit, and the scarf helps the adhesive to re-cure.

Another lace wig bone of contention is whether or not to disclose that you're wearing a wig, especially to your significant other. I don't understand why this has to be a secret. As much time as I spend on applications and the maintenance of my lace wigs, I can't imagine hiding it from my boyfriend. At first, there was that stigma of "ooh, I'm wearing a wig, I mustn't let anyone know". That first month of wearing the wig was torture for me, because I just knew everyone was looking at me. As my applications got better, my confidence level increased. I'm at the point now that it's no different than me just combing my hair. I know that some people want to keep it private and let it remain a mystery. Heaven forbid that you're sharing an intimate moment with your significant other, and your lace pops loose. That's a conversation I'm glad that I don't have to have. Maybe I'm lucky in that my boyfriend doesn't care one way or the other that I wear wigs; that he's evolved enough to realize that my hair is just an accessory, like makeup and clothes. He's been with me through my current hair journey (from shaved to curly), so he knows my wigs are just a means to an end (reaching my natural hair goal).

Once I shared my hair "hobby" with my boyfriend, I felt so much better about wearing the wigs. I can freely do an application in front of him, or remove my wig in front of him without having to sneak into the bathroom. When we go out, I always have him check my hairline to see if there is any "clownage" (adhesive showing). After that first moment of mortification early on, I saw that if I didn't make a big deal out of it, he wouldn't make a big deal out of it. Everyone has deal breakers, and if the fact that I wore wigs was a deal breaker for him, then he wouldn't be the guy for me. Luckily, he's the guy for me.

Don't be afraid to "get it on" while wearing your wig. As a movie going generation, we were raised on moments where the damsel in distress lures the hero in with her long flowing hair. Fast forward to modern times, it is now possible for us to flip and throw our hair just like Beyoncé and every other luxuriously long haired diva. Depending on what "level of application" I'm wearing, I have no fear of my hair clowning when intimate moments arise. More times than not, I'm usually wearing my headscarf, because that's where me and my boyfriend are with ours, but there are moments when my hair is looking fabulous, and my boyfriend happens to catch me in a mood where I don't want to wear my scarf. The next morning, I'm caught with that sexy bed head morning look. Those times aren't that often though, because I'm always wearing my scarf.

Sources of Information

It seems that beauty supply stores are now beginning to carry lace wigs and application supplies. I can't vouch for the quality of those wigs because I've never purchased a lace wig from the beauty supply store. More hair magazines are featuring sections about lace wigs also.

My source of information about lace wigs is the internet. That's where I started. There are many vendors, American and international, with websites offering any type of lace wig you want. Be warned that there are just as many people out there trying to scam you. Do the research, and shop around. Be warned of jumping on bandwagons also. They don't always work out.

There are many hair forums that have a lace wig section. I think the forums are a great place to learn, share, and fellowship with other lace wig wearers. I've developed a couple of good friendships by being a member of lace wig forums.

Some people are more visual than others (me included), and videos are helpful. YouTube is great source for lace wig education. I found Ms Lola on YouTube, and I'm so glad I did. I could see what she was doing, and it made more sense to me. Her voice is so soothing. I was inspired by Ms Lola, so I created quite a few lace wig tutorial videos and published them to YouTube. There are hundreds of lace wig videos on YouTube, all displaying different levels of knowledge and mastery. There is something out there for everyone.

I have become a source of information for some people. I wrote this book is a direct result of me opening up my YouTube email or regular email accounts and seeing ten to fifteen questions everyday. When I started on my lace wig odyssey, there wasn't a "how-to" lace wig manual. Hopefully with this book, I have provided it for you.

Purchasing Your First Lace Wig

The first thing to do before purchasing your first lace wig is to measure your head. There should be measurement information on the vendor's website. Some vendors visually show how to take the measurements, while some just have the stock measurements listed. With the permission of California Lace Wigs, I have provided their wig measurement guide at the end of this book (this information can be found on their website also).

There are so many elements to choose from when purchasing your first lace wig. This can be fun and frustrating, because sometimes, too much choice can be overwhelming. More than likely, you already know how you want your hair to look. My advice is to choose a straight or wavy texture (silky or kinky) for your first wig (either human or synthetic). Please don't choose a curly texture for your first wig. No matter what type of hair it's made with, a curly texture is a difficult texture to maintain. Don't say I didn't warn you.

There are many vendors to choose from. On the lace wig forums, a lot of members share their particular vendors, but there are some members who choose to keep their vendors secret. The reason being not to create a "rush" on that particular vendor, so the quality of the wigs will suffer. I don't necessarily agree with this non sharing theory, because it doesn't make sense that a vendor's quality of product would suffer because of an increase in business. The bread and butter of the international vendor's business are bulk orders. I don't think wigs from individual orders really affect an international vendor's business to the degree that their business should suffer. Word of mouth can be good or bad. I don't get into the politics of lace wigs. I recommend choosing a vendor and wig based on the wig you find that you like. I hate so say this, but because you can't see and touch the product before hand, you're taking a chance. I took a chance with both of my vendors, and they sent great product. There's no way you'll know what you're going to get, unless you order the wig. Unfortunately, it is a crapshoot.

The next thing to think about is whether you want a stock wig (a wig that the vendor has ready to ship) or a custom wig. Stock wigs usually ship very quickly, and you can receive them within a couple of days of the vendor receiving your payment. The speed of delivery depends on what shipping carrier the vendor uses. International vendors ship very quickly, which makes buying from an international vendor very attractive (along with the lower price). The payment and shipping information should be clearly stated on the vendor's website, unless it is an international vendor, in which you would have to request a current stock/price list.

Custom wigs are wigs that are custom made to your specifications. Anything you want, the sky's the limit (within the limitations of the particular vendor you choose). Custom wigs usually take weeks to make. The times vary from vendor to vendor. I've had several custom wigs made: a custom two toned colored wig; a texture added to virgin hair; an all lace wig without the PU strips covering the lace seams; some vendors carry stock wigs without the PU strips. My particular vendor doesn't.

After you decide on the wig you'd like to purchase, please study the vendor's website thoroughly. Make sure to read the return policy. You may want to establish contact with your vendor at this time, asking all the questions you need to ask before you send your money. If I'm ordering a stock wig, I'll ask my vendor if it's in stock, and for the price of the wig. If it's a custom, I'll email him my custom specifications and ask for the price and the shipping time.

Some vendors operate their websites just like an online store, and you add the products you want to your "cart" and "check out" by paying for your purchase with a credit or debit card. Other vendors require money transfers. Again, make sure you read and understand your vendor's payment and shipping policies before making your purchase.

Some people are wary about dealing with an international vendor. Most are based in China, as is my vendor. I've never had a problem sending money via Western Union or MoneyGram. Most international vendors also accept PayPal™. I've always received my wigs as promised also.

Okay, you've chosen your vendor, picked your wig, and paid your money. Now you play the waiting game. I think it's a lace wig phenomenon that once you order your wig, time stops. You're so excited that it's all you can think about. You begin to track your shipment as soon as your vendor emails your tracking number. Every time you hear a truck roll up, you run to the window, looking for the UPS man. A couple of days roll past. Finally, it's here! As I stated earlier, I was afraid of my first lace wig. Afraid I was going to damage it because it felt so delicate. I still get giddy when I receive a new wig. I digress. Back to you and your excitement.

You open the box or bag it came in. Usually, the American vendors package their wigs very nicely, with goodies like instructions on how to apply and remove the wig, a small wig brush, or comb, or hair care samples. It varies. Some vendors, like the international vendors, don't include anything but a hairnet and a label. All that matters is that the wig inside the plastic bag is the wig you ordered: the correct size, the correct color, and the correct length. Lucky for me, I haven't had to return a wig. I've had a wig that was misrepresented, but I loved it anyway and I made it work. I've heard some horror stories about people receiving the wrong wig, or not receiving their wig at all. There's always that chance when you order from anywhere other than a brick and mortar store.

When you open the box or bag, and you pull the wig out, it's exciting. Ah, the possibilities, of having the hair you've always wanted. Inspect the hair and inspect the lace, checking for any loose seams or bald spots. At this point, I suggest you pull on a wig cap and try the wig on to make sure it fits, and that you're happy with the hairline. If everything is okay, wash and condition the new wig with your favorite moisturizing shampoo and conditioner. Do not cut the lace at this point. By this time, if you haven't purchased a wig head (or mannequin head), now's the time to do so. If you've purchased a curly wig, I recommend laying it on a towel to let it dry. If you pin it to your wig head and let the hair hang, the weight of the hair may straighten the curls.

Lace Wig Supplies

Because there are several products that are a must in a lace wig supply kit, I will cover this topic in detail in Chapter 3. I want to stress that you will start off wanting to buy the "right" supplies – supplies found on your chosen vendor's website (if he/she sells them), or products raved about on various lace wig forums. More and more local beauty supply stores are beginning to carry lace wig adhesives and tapes. You will try a lot of products before you find which ones work for you. Don't be disappointed to find that the first adhesive you purchased doesn't work for you. Your body chemistry plays an important part in determining if the adhesive or tape will work for you. Also, be mindful of any allergic reactions. My nape seems to be allergic to Walker No-Shine A-Contour Tapes, so I use Supertape™ Thin Sticks™ for my nape and the Walker tapes for my front hairline (from temples to sideburns). Please be aware of physical reactions you may have, as you're dealing with chemicals.

Cutting the Lace

Once the wig is dry, try it on again. If it is too small, you will have to send it back to the vendor. I don't recommend that you try to add to it if you are a newbie. If it is too big, you can always sew a seam in the back of the wig to make it fit. If the fit is good, it's time to cut the lace. The very first time you do this will be nerve wrecking. My early research lead to me buying pinking shears (scissors with the zigzag blades). They're still new in the package. Maybe the ones I purchased were too big, but I've never used them. I use small, very sharp scissors, and I make small snips as close to the hairline as I can get, all around the lace. I don't leave any lace. Sometimes, I clip a little into the hairline, especially on the temples and sideburns, to make the hairline look as realistic as possible. Be careful when cutting your hairline. You don't want to cut the dreaded moon shape across the hairline – that's automatic advertising that you're wearing a lace wig. This is why it is advised that when you measure for your wig, you allow for ¼ of an inch beyond (in front of) your actual hairline, so the lace can lay on your skin and not on your actual hair, and you can cut a more realistic hairline.

As with anything dealing with lace wigs, the more you do it, the easier it gets. The key is taking your time and slowly clipping as close to the hairline as you can get. For those who need it, there is a video of me cutting the lace on a new wig, on my YouTube channel.

Bleaching the Knots

Once you cut the lace, there are things you can do to enhance the realistic appearance of the wig. You can cover or color the knots (the point where the hair is tied onto the lace). Unbleached knots resemble a crop of ants resting on top of your head – not a good look. Some people use hair bleach to lighten the color of the knots. Virgin hair knots lift quite easily. The knot bleaching stage always reveals whether the vendor has used fabric dye on the hair to achieve the darker colors (black, off black, and dark brown). If the color doesn't lift with the bleach, then it has been dyed with fabric dye. To combat this issue, you will need to use a fabric dye remover. This can be very tricky, because as I stated earlier, the dye remover can alter the color (obviously) and the texture of the hair. Once the hair has been dipped (lace only), the knots should be light enough.

Bleaching knots can be effective, but I don't condone it, because although it makes the hair look like it's growing from the scalp, it makes the knots weak, and weak knots cause the hair to shed. I know this from personal experience. I once bleached knots on a couple of my favorite wigs, and although it looked natural, the hair began to shed, so much that on one of the wigs, it became unwearable. Lesson learned: find a new way to cover my knots, without ruining my wigs. There are instructions on the internet explaining the knot bleaching methods. Please be careful if you decide to bleach your knots using hair bleach and developer.

Scalp Techniques

Along with bleaching/coloring the knots, achieving a realistic scalp is a great technique to learn. There are various methods used by different people. You may start off using one technique, and find something else that works even better.

For my scalp technique, I start off with a scalp colored (tan) wig cap, found at my local beauty supply store. You can also use tan colored panty hose or a knee-hi stocking to achieve the same effect. I use the wig cap to protect my braided hair from the lace. I used to use leg makeup spray (along with a blonde highlighting spray) to cover my knots and simulate a scalp, but I found that method to be too orange for my skin tone. There is a fake knot bleaching video on my YouTube channel, demonstrating this method. It still works for some people. Try it and see. The great thing about lace wigs is that none of these techniques are written in stone, and once you become a wearer, you begin to discover better ways to achieve the "holy grail" of the lace wig – a flawless application. I digress. Back on topic...

I've recently discovered the wonders of painting either my wig cap or the inside of my lace with regular drugstore liquid foundation makeup. I customize the color by mixing several different shades to closely match the color of my scalp. I use a large foundation brush and I lightly paint the inside of the lace. Make sure not to paint too heavily. If you paint it on and it comes through the lace, wipe it off with alcohol and a paper towel. Be sure to let it dry for at least fifteen minutes. I also seal it with my clear acrylic sealant spray.

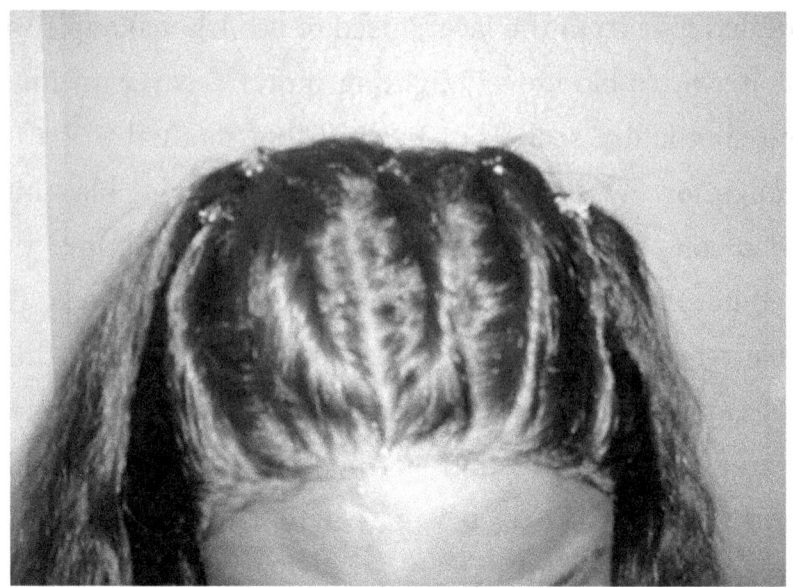

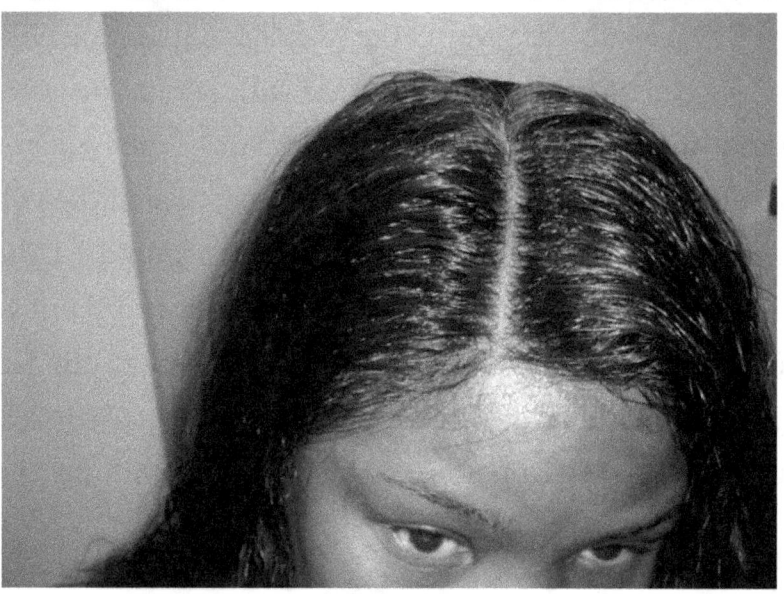

Another method for achieving a realistic looking scalp is to use a self adhesive bandage, readily found in drugstores and any place that sells bandages. I tried to use it two years ago with my first application, but I couldn't get the hang of it. This was one method in which I needed a visual tutorial in order to understand. I finally found a YouTube video in which the person really took her time and explained what she was doing. I got it. I've been using the bandage method ever since (thanks MsShayelove). With the bandage method, you can basically recreate a new hairline, provided you're able to match the color of the bandage to your complexion, and the bandage doesn't show past the lace edge. I combine the wig cap with the bandage wrap for the most protection of my hair and my natural hairline. Using the bandage method with my makeup method gives me the most realistic looking scalp.

Application Techniques

There are several ways you can apply your lace wig. Adhesive by itself, tape by itself, adhesive and tape together, wig clips, hair pins, and bobby pins. Some people remove their wigs daily, while others opt to wear their wigs for longer periods of time (like myself). Sometimes I'll attach the front with adhesive and tape, and attach the back of my wig with wig clips. Find what works for you, and perfect it.

Shedding/Sealing the Knots

Shedding can be the kiss of death for a wig. It can result from bleaching the knots, over-processing the hair (from coloring and texturizing), brushing too vigorously, or from poor ventilating (the process of hand tying the hair onto the lace). The only shedding I've experienced is due from bleaching the knots. Some would argue that using the correct bleaching method shouldn't affect the strength of the knots, but I beg to differ. Any chemical that breaks down the molecular structure of the hair will cause the hair to shed. Please be careful with any extra processing of the hair. To combat shedding, you must seal your knots.

You should always seal the knots on the wig after every washing, and especially after bleaching the knots. This means to turn the wig inside out and spray the lace with a clear acrylic sealant. This is to protect the knots from becoming loose. This spray can be found in any craft store, or any store that has a craft section. Most home building supply stores should carry the sealant also (don't laugh). You can also use a heavy duty hairspray (Schwarzkoppf's göt2b glued blasting Freeze Spray is what I use). Please let the sealant dry for at least fifteen minutes before applying your wig. I also seal the lace after I paint the makeup onto the lace. It may take a couple washings to get the makeup off your lace, but this will not damage the lace.

Bleach Bath

A bleach bath is a two step bleach and ammonia process used to detangle or de-puff a human hair wig. Luckily for me, I've never had to do a bleach bath on any of my wigs. Please search the internet for instructions and videos on how to do this. Since I've never done it, I don't feel qualified to instruct you on how to do it.

Thinning a Lace Wig

If you find that your wig is thicker than you'd like, you can lessen the density of your wig. Many people use thinning shears to do this. I purchased a pair of thinning shears to use on my first Indian Remy Kinky Curly wig (from Rex), but I never got around to it because I killed the wig. The thinning shears (or blending shears) have teeth on one blade and the other blade is a regular cutting blade. You clip close to the lace, preferably underneath the top layer of the hair, so the little hairs left over won't poke through the hair. Again, there are many wig thinning videos on YouTube.

My Moments of Mortification

I guess I'm lucky in that I've never had a bad public lace wig situation. As I stated earlier, my most horrific public moment of mortification was in the third month of wearing lace wigs, and that moment really wasn't so bad.

My boyfriend didn't see the liftage or the white ring caused by my hairline getting wet.

Another bad lace wig moment was when I tried to bleach the knots on my favorite 18 inch Virgin Malaysian loose curly wig. I loved that wig. The knots weren't as light as I needed them to be. I still wasn't good at bleaching knots, but how does one learn, right? So I got my bleaching supplies, and began painting the cap. Since the hair was so dark, I didn't think the color would lift so fast, but lift it did, within five minutes. I panicked because, of course, the section I first started in was more blonde than the section I finished last. The bleach bled through to the roots, so my roots were orange and blonde, on a 1B unit – not a good look at all. I was crushed, because I loved that wig. After getting myself together, I researched ways to fix my mess. Another trip to the beauty supply store for hair color and a highlighting wand (they practically know me by my name). It painstakingly took two hours to color in the orangey blonde roots. The sad thing is that I had to retire the wig because it began to shed. This mishap led me to my new method of painting my knots with my custom makeup blend.

I've heard some really bad horror stories: lace wigs sliding back to reveal tape and adhesive; being pulled down a bed and having your wig almost slide off your head (also happened to me); a lace wig stealing pet; someone talking to you and looking directly at your head for the whole conversation – there are millions of horror stories. Just as there are many bad stories, there are millions of good stories and all of them have one thing in common – that it involved a flawless application. As it's said many times, I'll say it again: the more you apply your lace wigs, the better you'll get, if you're open to learn, listen, read and research. I still have bad apps from time to time. I deal with it and hope that the next application will be better.

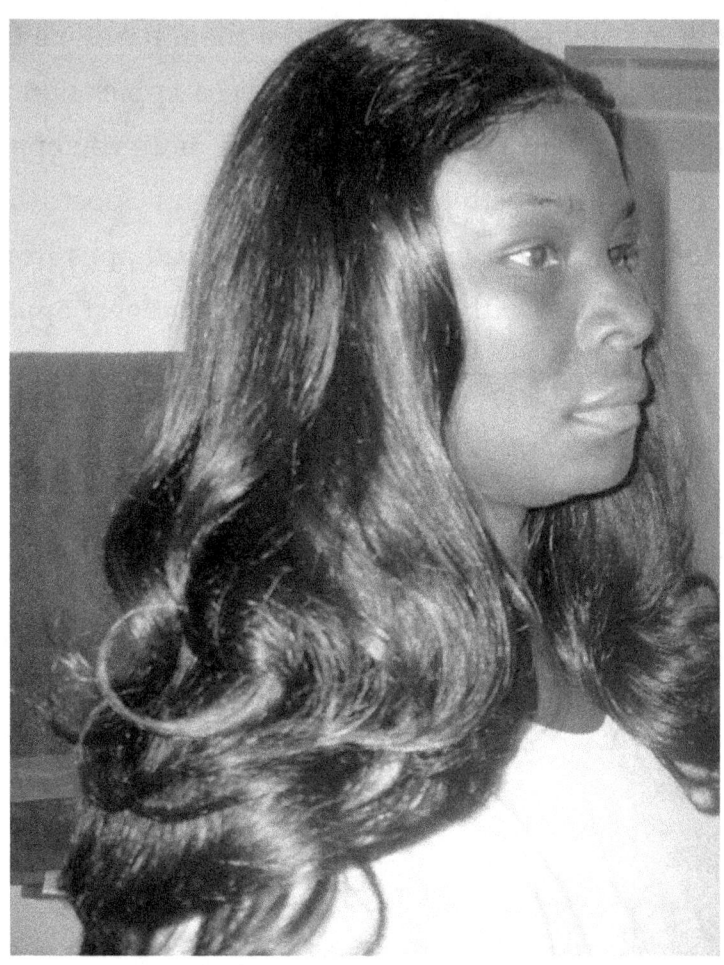

20 inch virgin Indian straight/wavy (CLW)

Chapter 3

My Lace Wigs Tutorials

Now's the time to roll up your sleeves and get to work. It will be hard for some, scary for others, and frustrating for most. It gets easier and quicker as you do more applications. Every now and then, you'll have a bad app; I still do. Don't sweat it. It happens. Just mentally note where you went wrong so you'll know what not to do the next time.

Gathering Your Supplies

The most important tool in my lace wig supplies kit is my digital camera. I have taken pictures of every app I've ever done, not because I'm narcissistic, but because photos are a good way to document your progress. I recommend purchasing one if you don't already have one.

My Current Lace Wig Supply List:

Supertape™ Thin Sticks™

Walker No-Shine A-Contour Tapes

Vapon NOTAPE® Silicone Bonding Adhesive, 1 oz tube

HD White Adhesive

Endura-Bond™ (hard bond) Adhesive

Tan wig caps or knee-hi nylons; brown weaving thread

Self Adhering bandage in tan

Wooden craft sticks (for applying the adhesive)

Lighted mirror and hand mirror (for applying the nape)

Scissors (hair cutting and manicure for the small snips)

Q-Tips (for hairline clean ups)

Towel

Rattail comb

Wide tooth comb,

A brush with round edged bristles, or a Looper brush

Tweezers

Hair clips (to clip the baby hairs back when applying the wig)

FabricMate™ Marker, in Brown or Tan, to color the lace

Foundation makeup (the color of your scalp)

Large foundation brush (to paint the makeup on)

Clear acrylic spray sealant (found at the craft store)

<u>My removal supplies:</u>

Oil sheen (any brand, but I use Motions in the yellow can)

91% or 99% alcohol

100% pure acetone

Goo Gone® Spray Gel

Creamy conditioner or face cream (Ponds)

Repair supplies:

Clear thread (found at any fabric store);

Sewing needles;

Scissors

Fray block™

Supplies to Carry In Your Purse:

Cover Grey Stick in the color of your wig hair

FabricMate pen in the color of your wig hair

White Adhesive (for emergency pop ups)

Endura-Bond

Wooden craft sticks

I've gone through several products to finally find the ones that work for me. Pay attention to how your body reacts to your adhesives. The Walker tapes make my nape break out but not my hairline (as I stated earlier). I love Supertape but not for my hairline (because it can be seen through the lace). Hopefully, you have the patience to find out the right combination for you. As you can see, there is no hard and fast rule when it comes to lace wigs. These are guidelines, but you have to find what works for you.

I only use Endura-Bond in emergency situations, when I'm out and my wig wants to clown. It's rare that I have to break it out, but I always carry it with me just in case. I always use it on top of tape, and only use a very thin layer, sticking the lace down immediately. You do not wait for the Endura-Bond to cure, and I recommend using it directly on top of tape and not your skin. It's similar to super glue, so be careful with it.

I also will cover my clownage with whatever I have in my purse, be it brown lip stain or eyeliner... anything to cover the tale-tale grayish-white edges that want to surface at the wrong times. Unorthodox, I know, but it does the trick. This is only when I'm out in public and I see white at my hairline.

Prepping Your Hair

Make sure the area you're working in is well ventilated. It helps to have everything laid out in the order that you're going to use it. Before you start, I recommend you start with a clean wig, with the knots already sealed. To get a great app, you have to make your own hair as flat as you can get it. Depending on how long your own hair is, you can have it braided or wrapped. When I first started wearing lace wigs, I used to have my sister braid my hair. Eventually, I learned how to cornrow my own hair, thanks to YouTube. Soon after, I let the wrong person give me a jacked up haircut, which caused me to shave my head bald. When my head was shaved, I had the best apps. My head was smooth underneath, and there were no braid bumps. As my hair grew out, I continued to shave my nape to help the lace stick but I don't do this anymore. I don't recommend this practice at all. My hair has grown back out, even longer than when I started wearing lace wigs, in just two years.

For the longest time, I didn't wear a wig cap underneath my lace, but now I do, to protect my hair. I sew the wig cap onto my braids so it doesn't slide back, then I cut the band off of the cap, pretty close to the braid.

My current braiding pattern, front

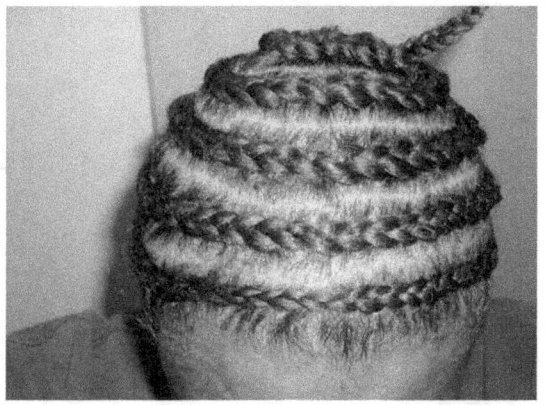

My current braiding pattern, top

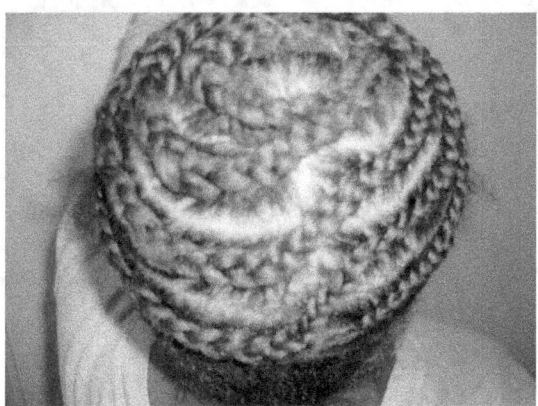

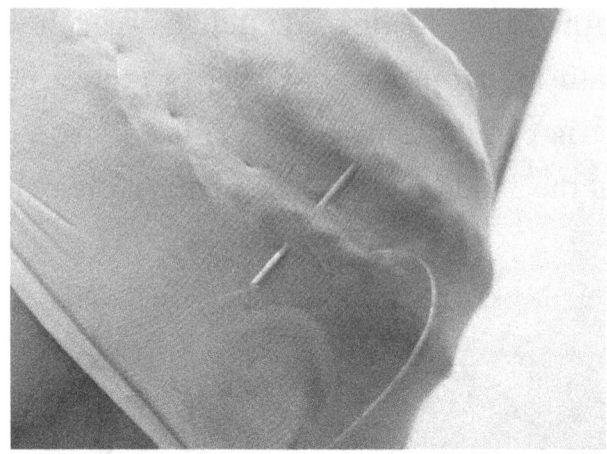

Above: sewing the wig cap onto my braids.

Below: cutting the band off the wig cap.

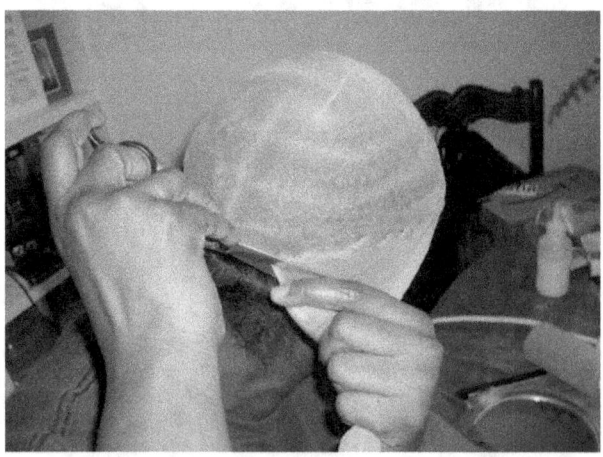

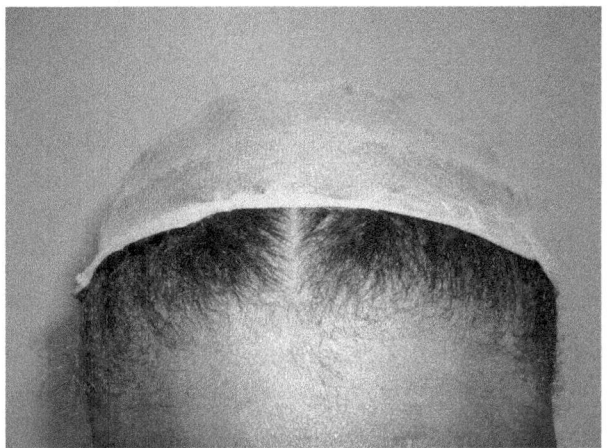

The wig cap sewn on.

Prepping Your Hairline

After I sew the wig cap to my braid and cut the band off, I wipe the entire circumference of my hairline with a hand towel and 91% or 99% alcohol two or three times, and I let my skin dry completely. Some people use a skin protectant, but I don't. I used to, but I found that it left a white ring around my hairline. I find that my adhesives are gentle enough on my skin for me to skip this step. If you do choose to use a skin protectant, please use one or two thin layers, and let it dry completely before proceeding to the next step.

Using the Self Adhering Bandage Method

On one of the forums I'm a member of, some of the members with the most fierce apps use the self adhering bandage method. For the longest time, I couldn't, for the life of me, figure out how they were wrapping their heads with it. They would explain and explain, but I couldn't get it. I remember buying a bandage early on, and just staring at it, like "how is this going to work?" I never used it; in fact, I sent it to another member for free! Fast forward to a year (and a couple of months) later. I found MsShaylove's video on the bandage wrap method, and she made it look so easy. So I followed her instructions, and voila! My hairline was wrapped. I'm getting good at it now. I prefer four inch wide bandages, but I'm not particular on any specific brand. I love how the bandage covers as much of my hairline as it can. I've started sewing the ends of the bandage together to make a headband, so I don't have to worry about the bandage unraveling under my lace. Depending on what color the bandage is, I may brush my custom makeup foundation blend over it, letting it dry completely before moving to the next step. If you get any makeup on your skin, please clean it off with the alcohol before continuing.

Laying the Tape

During my first year wearing lace wigs, my apps frustrated me because by the second or third day, the lace would begin to slide back on my head. The adhesive would melt due to the changes in my body temperature. I adopted the 'tape first' method suggested to me by fellow

BHM forum member LuvMyHair631. I'm sure other people use this method, and I'm not saying she invented it, but she suggested it to me. With that ass-covering disclosure aside, this is how I do it. I'm offering two methods, the nape method, which I don't use anymore because my nape hair is too long (and I don't want to keep shaving my nape); and the part method, which is a bit controversial. If you're going to adhere the lace to your nape (past your hairline), I don't see any other way around shaving your nape up a bit.

For the front of my head, I put wide strips of the Walker No-Shine Tape from my temple to my sideburn (on both sides; leave the center of the forehead tape free). I leave the tape wide so half can lay on my skin and the other half can lay on the bandage. Eventually you will be able to gauge how far back you should start your bandage and your tape. Using the bandage gives you an opportunity to create a whole new hairline, if you can get the bandage to blend into your complexion.

Since the bandage is covering my entire head, I line the entire edge of the bandage with the Walker No-Shine Tape all the way around. This gives me the most secure feeling application.

<u>Nape method</u>: On each side of my head, behind my ears, I place a strip of the Supertape Thin Sticks along the length of my nape. Then I lay the strips across my nape, under my hairline:

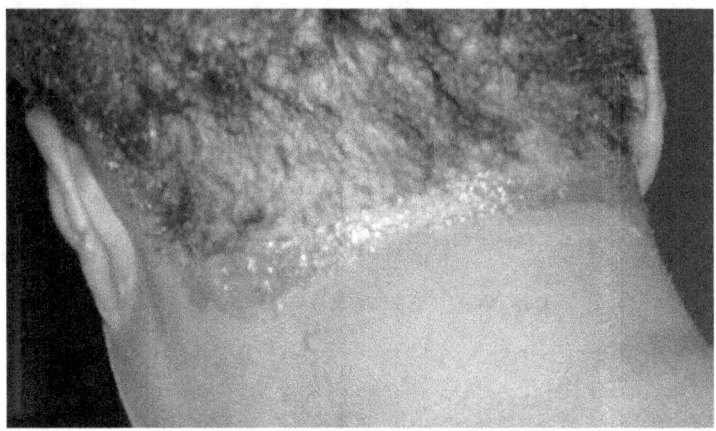

This method worked quite well, when I used to shave my nape. I don't use this method anymore, because I'm letting all of my hair grow out.

<u>Part method</u>: Since my hair has grown out, I leave my nape out. I make a part about two inches up from my nape and section it off with a rubber band. I cut a strip of the Supertape in half lengthwise and I lay it right on my part, then I lay the bandage on the tape. This secures the back:

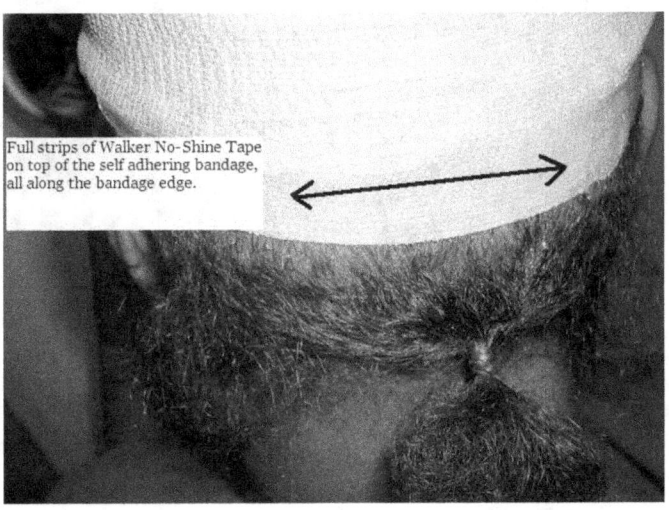

Full strips of Walker No-Shine Tape on top of the self adhering bandage, all along the bandage edge.

I know, at this point, you're saying, "what the hell?" Stay with me here! I don't like for my hair to pull at the nape. There is no way I can have the nape of my wigs sitting so far down past the hairs on my neck, and again, I'm not shaving my nape anymore. I rarely wear high ponytails in public, but I'm still able to wear ponytails if I want to.

Not meaning to jump the gun, but I'm going to show you the after picture, so you can understand what I did:

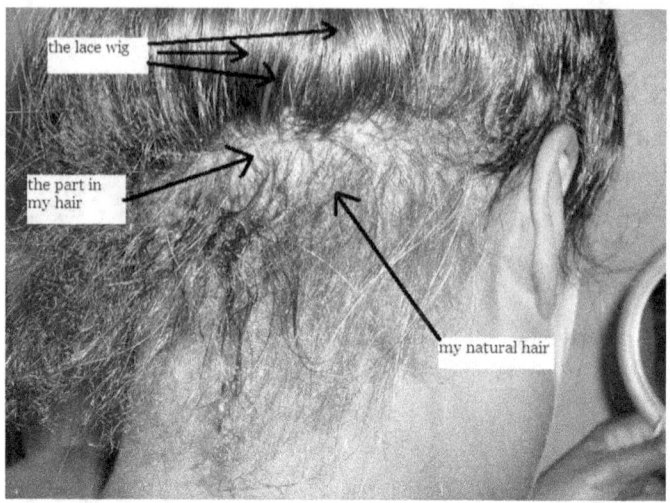

I may be biased, but I can hardly see where the lace wig stops and my real hair starts. If you want, you can sew wig clips into your wig edge, and secure the wig that way. This would mean cutting your wig up to this point, or ordering custom wigs with this forehead-to-upper nape measurement. This is the method I'm using right now.

Applying the Adhesive

<u>10-day hold (level 2)</u>:

1. Vapon – 15 minutes drying time
2. Vapon – 15 minutes drying time
3. White Adhesive – 10 minutes drying time

<u>+10-day hold (level 3)</u>:

1. Vapon – 15 minutes drying time
2. Vapon – 15 minutes drying time
3. Vapon – 15 minutes drying tome
4. White adhesive – 10 minutes drying time

This next step is made easier by the previous step. The tape provides an even guide on which to spread the adhesive. I start off with the first layer of my favorite silicone adhesive, Vapon NOTAPE® Silicone Bonding adhesive, in the one ounce tube. Many people find Vapon to be messy; use the silicone adhesive you that gives you the best hold. For me, the key to working with Vapon is squeezing out an amount the size of the head of a thumbtack on to a wooden craft stick. Spread it until there is no more on the stick. Repeat the squeezing and spreading until all of the tape is covered. Try not to overlap on the wet areas. Make sure you replace the cap or top back onto the tube or container of your adhesive. Let this layer dry for fifteen minutes. While this layer is drying, you could line the inside edge of your lace in the nape area with thin strips of tape (the key to a non lifting nape).

After the first fifteen minutes, it's time for another layer of the Vapon (or your silicone adhesive), following the same squeezing and spreading technique above. Replace the cap on the adhesive. Let this layer dry for another fifteen minutes.

Now this is what I mean by "level of application", mentioned back in Chapter 2. If I stop at the second layer of silicone adhesive, this would be a ten day application, with maybe a minor touch-up on a random edge on day 8 or 9. This is my everyday app (including the white adhesive later). If you're traveling and you want to feel a little bit more secure, I recommend adding a third layer of silicone adhesive (Vapon for me), again letting it dry for fifteen minutes. This third layer took me past fourteen days (during which I went to Mexico, with no reapplication).

Whether you stop at "level 2" or "level 3" with your silicone adhesive, the last layer you will need is the white adhesive layer. Hair Direct White Adhesive (HDWA) is the only white adhesive that works for me, but use what works for you. I use a new wooden craft stick to spread the white adhesive over the silicone layers. I extend it a millimeter outside of the silicone edge. I let this dry for 10 minutes, or until clear.

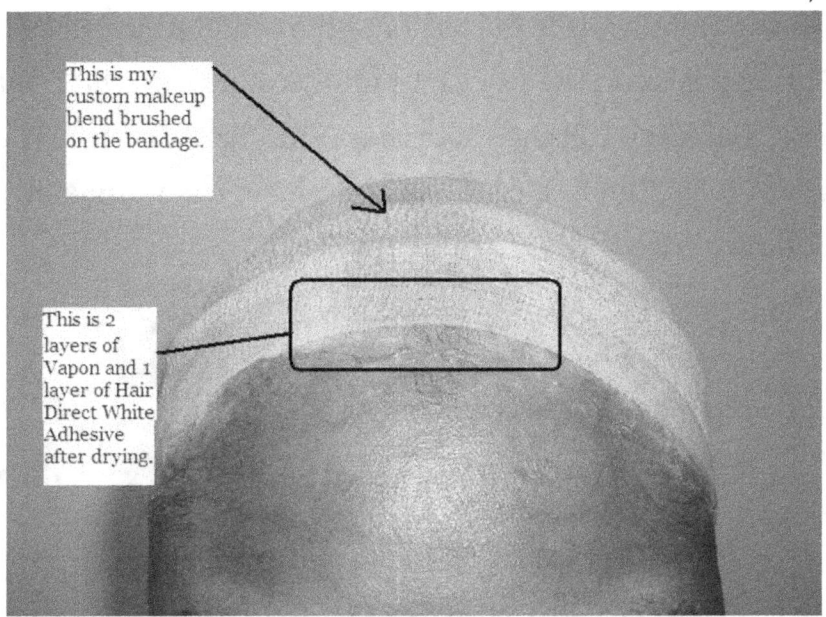

The white adhesive takes down the shine of the silicone adhesive layers. I've been using it since my very first application. Although there are baby hairs in the adhesive, this is the exact placement for the bandage/adhesive, in order for my applications to look natural. If the bandage is too far forward, it wouldn't look natural. The Goo Gone Gel Spray gently removes any adhesive from my hairline.

Applying the Lace Wig

Finally! Well, almost. I'm sure, if you're a newbie reading this, and you're at this step, you're quite nervous. That's understandable. Breathe... and then breathe again.

Make sure your wig is clipped or rolled back onto itself, exposing the lace. Make sure all baby hair is clipped back. Carefully place the wig onto the center of your head, letting it rest on the wig cap. I always start with the front first. Carefully roll the center edge into the adhesive. The key is to get the lace edge as close as you can to the outer adhesive edge:

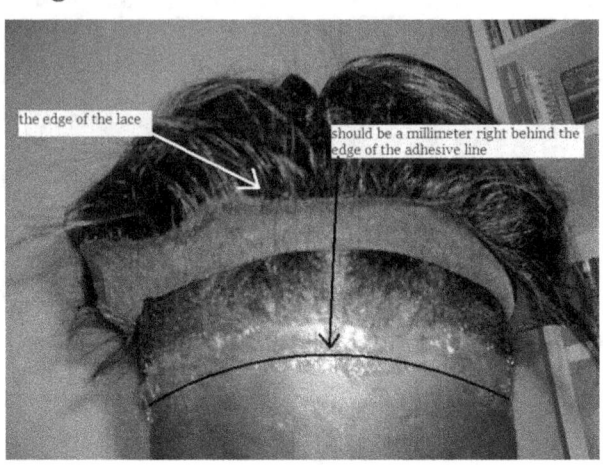

the edge of the lace

should be a millimeter right behind the edge of the adhesive line

You want to get the edge of the lace as close to the adhesive edge as you can, so you won't have that much adhesive, if any, to clean off your forehead. Press the lace into the adhesive with a comb, preferably a small tooth comb. Do not use your fingers because the oils on your fingers may seep through the lace and reduce the tack of the adhesive. Repeat this all along the front edge, on both sides, making sure to take your time. Check to make sure that your temples and sideburns are even. Do not pull on your lace to make these areas even. If you have to pull to make it fit, then you've either ordered a wig too small, or you've cut too much when trimming the lace or customizing your hairline. The lace should naturally fall in front of where your temples and sideburns are, which should hit right above where your ear starts.

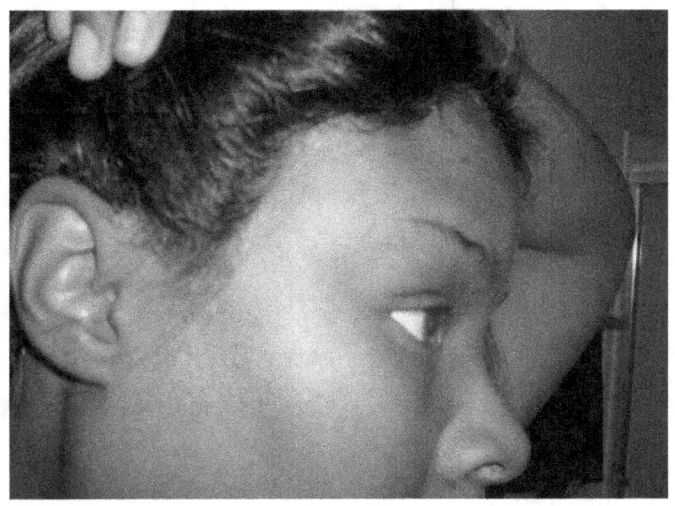

Notice how the wig hairline curves around from my forehead to my temples. Don't be afraid to customize your hairline, because rarely does a stock lace wig look good enough to put on right out of the bag.

Once you get the front secured and bonded, it's time to do the back. For those who are dexterous, eventually you will be able look at the back of your head through tabletop mirror (in my case, a lighted mirror) while you're holding your hand mirror and rolling your lace down. I've had years of practice doing the back of my hair, either curling or braiding my own hair.

Carefully pull the paper tabs off the tape on the nape lace (with tweezers if you need them). If your nape lace is measured and cut correctly, you can start at either end. With your chin resting downward (like you're looking at the floor), carefully line up the lace edge with the edge of the adhesive on your nape. Turn your head to the right, and attach the left side of the nape. Go slowly, because the lace will want to fold onto itself, and if that happens, you'll pull the tape off the nape of the lace. This has happened to me many times. Okay, once you get one edge down, slowly move across the nape, lining the lace edge up with the adhesive edge. Do the same for the right side, turning your head to the left. Be sure to use your comb to work the lace into the adhesive. Don't forget to press the lace into the adhesive behind the ears also.

After successfully attaching the lace to your perimeter, now you can take your fingers and feel around your perimeter to make sure all the edges are down. You may feel a little adhesive on the edge. This is actually a good thing. You can rub your baby hairs into that excess adhesive to give your edges a more natural look. In the event there are some edges that didn't attach, use a clean craft stick and smooth a little bit of the white adhesive on the area. Let dry until clear, and comb the lace down. Repeat rubbing your edges down and arranging the baby hair.

I find that when I use this method, I have very little adhesive to clean off my hairline. If there is adhesive to clean, I use 91% or 99% alcohol on a cotton swab and wipe the adhesive until it disappears, without touching the lace edge. If any alcohol gets on the edge, it may cause the lace to lift.

I hear a lot of people complaining about how their napes won't stay down. In my experience, putting the tape on the nape edge of the lace (along with the tape and adhesive on your skin) will give you a nape that will not budge. It does take practice (without looking) to lift the paper tabs off of the tape without the edge catching onto the tape and sticking to itself. Then you have to re-line the lace edge with the tape, while the front is still on your head.

Once you've done a perimeter check to make sure all the lace edges are buried in the adhesive, and you've cleaned your hairline of all excess adhesive, you can tie a scarf around your hairline as tight as you can stand. I prefer to do applications in the evening, so I can keep my hair tied down all night long, in order to achieve the tightest bond.

Excluding gathering my supplies, prepping my hair and wig, my applications take as long as the amount of adhesive layers that need to dry. I don't trip off of how long it takes to lay tape around my perimeter. Thirty minutes is enough time for a light layer of sealant or heavy duty hairspray to dry (for knot spraying, if you haven't done so beforehand) before applying your wig. Pick an off day to spend on doing an application. I can't imagine doing an app right before going to work or going to an event. Sometimes my boyfriend will want to go somewhere right when I've finished an app, and I can't immediately tie it down. If my app clowns, he knows where I'm placing the blame!

As I stated earlier, my "level 2" app lasts about ten days, depending on how long I can stand it. Sometimes I take it off before then, or I'll let it stay on longer. The adhesive begins to itch a little bit around the hairline between day 8 and day 9. I wash my wigs on my head at least twice during my apps. I try to never get my scalp wet, but if I do, I'll sit under a hooded hairdryer to make sure my braids dry completely. There is also a hair freshener available for those who suffer from sweaty scalps. It's available at your local drugstore.

The worst clownage I see is my front edges lifting around day 7 or 8. I keep my white adhesive handy so I can run a bead of adhesive on the edge of a wooden craft stick and put it on the exposed area, let dry until clear, then stick the lace back down, and keep it moving. The more I learn, the less drastic the clownage is. The key is to know when it's time to remove your application.

The most important key to a great long lasting application is tying it down every night with a silk or satin scarf. The nightly tying down allows for the adhesive to re-bond overnight.

Removal of the Wig

The dreaded removal day. I hate removal day. Sometimes, I wish I could just let the wig walk off my head by itself. Just like my application techniques, my removal techniques have evolved into a more health friendly, "find it locally" approach. When I first started, I used to remove my apps with PURE Citru-spice ™ Adhesive Remover, purchased from my first vendor. It was oily and it smelled lovely; but I'm a "get it from around the corner" kind of girl; many hours of research led me to learn that 100% acetone (nail polish remover) could be used to cut through the silicone adhesive layers. I could readily get the acetone at my local beauty supply store. I immediately found out that acetone was strictly for soaking the wig in*, as it practically burned the skin off of my forehead. Lesson learned. More research pointed me to Goo Gone® Spray (either liquid or gel). I like the way Goo Gone foams up. The key to removing your application is PATIENCE. This is the point where many hairlines have been lost. This is what I do:

I begin by wrapping a towel around my neck, because this will be messy. I spray my entire hairline with alcohol (either 91% or 99% in a spray bottle) to soften the adhesive. Then I spray the Goo Gone onto the hairline, saturating it. I make sure to wipe my face periodically, as the alcohol and Goo Gone will run; you don't want to get any of the solution in your eyes. Once I saturate my hairline, I begin to rub my hairline, working the Goo Gone into a sudsy foam. I keep doing this until the lace begins to lift from my skin. Sometimes the adhesive and tape separate from the lace and remain on my skin. If that happens, I make sure to keep rubbing until the lace completely releases the tape. DO NOT PULL THE LACE FROM YOUR SKIN!!! If you do, you will tear the lace. Let whatever removal solvent you use do the work for you.

Once the lace releases from my head, I spray the inside of the lace (where the adhesive and tape was) with the Goo Gone, and sit the wig in the sink. I spray more Goo Gone onto my hairline, and rub until the adhesive and tape comes off. This can take a couple of hours. I am in no rush, as I'm trying to preserve my hairline. I find that Goo Gone is very gentle on my hair, as long as I let it do its job and not force it. When my hairline is as clean as I can get it, I use facial cleanser on a cotton pad to clean up the area. I follow that step up with slathering my hairline with a creamy hair conditioner, until I'm able to wash my hair.

Once my hairline is free of adhesive and tape, I either wash my hair with my braids intact (if I'm immediately doing another app after my hair dries), or I take my braids down and give my hair and scalp a thorough cleansing, depending on how long the I kept the braids in. While I'm walking around the house with my hair full of shampoo, I check on my wig, to see if the Goo Gone has dissolved all the adhesive gunk on the wig. I take an old (clean) toothbrush and gently brush away any adhesive that's left. This step usually takes about thirty minutes. Once I inspect the entire surface of the lace and make sure that there's no adhesive left, I rinse it with lukewarm water, and then I begin the shampoo process. I only soak the edges of the wig in acetone if the adhesive has not dissolved per my instructions above.

*I do not recommend using acetone to clean wigs with polyurethane (thin skin, PU strips). The acetone will weaken and/or eat away at the polyurethane. Acetone can eat through plastic, so do not keep acetone in plastic bottles. You should only use acetone in glass containers.

Washing the Wig

With the wig inside out (with the lace showing), I hold the wig with one hand, and in the other hand, I pour a capful of shampoo onto the wig. I've always used TRESemmé® Vitamin E Moisture Rich Shampoo and Conditioner on my wigs. It's very reasonably priced, I can find it at my local drugstore, and I love the way it makes the hair feel. By all means, use whatever moisture shampoos and conditioners you like, but make sure they're moisture restorers. Remember, lace wig hair lacks moisture because the hair has been cut from its moisture source.

I make sure I clean the perimeter of the lace, inside and out. There may be little globs of adhesive in the hair around the adhesive edge, so you want to pay special attention to that area. Do not scrub hard, and try not to rub the hair against itself. Just take your thumb and forefinger and lightly rub the area on the lace.

After I clean the perimeter and lace edge, I hold the wig up and I slide the suds down to the ends of the hair. You can finger comb the hair if needed to keep it from tangling. After I do this a couple of times, I rinse the wig in cool water until all the suds are gone. I pour a cap full of the conditioner onto the hair, and I comb it through with a wide tooth comb. I leave the conditioner on the hair for two to three minutes. Then I rinse in cool water. While the hair is dripping, I lay it in a towel, and squeeze the towel, which draws the water from the hair. Once most of the water is gone, I put the wig onto the mannequin head with T-pins and comb the hair straight. If the hair is wavy or curly, I still pin the wig to the mannequin head, but I brush the hair with my Denman brush. Then I place the head on a surface like a dresser or a floor on top of a towel, and I bunch the hair around the base of the mannequin head. Doing it this way ensures that the curls or waves stay springy. Always make sure your wig is dry before reapplying it. Many lace wig wearers have more than one wig to wear, in order to rotate for cleaning. This also lengthens the life of your wigs, because you're not wearing just one wig constantly. It's your choice, of course.

Caring for/Storing Your Lace Wig

There was once a time when I had more than 10 lace wigs. I kept them in a plastic container with a lid (in case of a flood). I kept each wig stuffed with its tissue paper, covered in its hairnet, and in the plastic bag it originally arrived in. On the outside of the bags, I wrote the type and length of wig. I've since sold all but four of my wigs (I will address lace wig addiction in a later chapter). One has been permanently retired (a hybrid of two of my favorite wigs that now sheds incessantly), another one has a bald spot in the back (that I will practice my ventilating skills on), and two are in current rotation, a straight wig and a curly wig (which needs major work – I cut the bangs too short*). I have three Styrofoam mannequin heads that I got from my local beauty supply store, along with three head holders (the kind that clamp onto a table), and wig T-pins. There are times when I don't feel like immediately cleaning a wig after I take it off. I want to put it in a plastic bag and hang it behind the bathroom door. I force myself to clean my wigs and store them properly, since I only have a few in my stash, and I want those to last as long as they can. Create the good habits now, and it pays off in the end. It would suck to take off a wig, and because you didn't feel like cleaning the other one, there wasn't a clean wig to put on.

*I cut the bangs too short on the curly wig, so I decided to use the hair to ventilate the future wigs I'm going to make.

Coloring the Lace

Vendors offer a variety of lace colors, from transparent to dark brown. I've had transparent (too light for my complexion), but I mainly get light brown lace (the lace color of my vendor's stock wigs). My advice is to try to match as close to your complexion as possible. If you receive a wig and the lace is not the color you need it to be, you can dye it with a fabric dye, i.e., Rit Dye, which comes in mixable colors. Experiment with different colors to find the shade you like.

Just as quick as you can dye the lace, you can also remove the dye, with a fabric dye remover (Rit Dye Remover). Follow the mixing directions, and <u>dip your unit in and out of the solution</u>, until you see the solution change colors (may turn yellowish). Do not soak your lace in the solution. Watch the hair carefully to see if it changes. Be careful if you decide you need to do this. The fabric dye remover will alter the hair texture and color.

Some people use the fabric dye remover to lighten their knots instead of bleaching them. Use caution, please, if you decide to use the dye remover. Please read the instructions.

Coloring the Hair

Okay, this is different from the previous "Hair Color" section. I'm talking about you changing the color of the hair, instead of ordering it already colored from the vendor. This can be fun, but also scary, if you don't know what you're doing. I've had experience from coloring my own hair, so when it came time to start coloring my units, there was no fear.

If you bleach your knots, unless you're a bleaching genius, the bleach may bleed onto your roots (remember my horror story). An easy fix! Buy a box of hair color (or color and developer — a tad complicated), and a highlighting brush (it looks like a extra large mascara wand, or better yet, just use an old, clean mascara wand). You can get in really close to the lace and brush the color onto the blonde parts. Leave it on per the instructions, rinse out well, deep condition, rinse, and let dry - all fixed.

You can experiment with different color combinations, or mix your favorite custom color. I love the two toned look, where the roots are dark, and the color lightens towards the ends of the hair. Or as I stated earlier, I like to bleach individual strands on my curly wigs. This is an area where you can be totally creative. I spray hair lightener (with lemon) onto my virgin Malaysian straight and let the sun naturally lighten it. It looks more natural to me.

Repairing Your Lace Wig

There will be a time when your wig will require type of repair: sewing up a hole, resizing the lace, or adding hair. Don't freak out. It's easy to take care of. Make sure your lace wig supply kit includes: clear thread (found at any craft or fabric store); sewing needles; scissors; and Fray Block™. Fray Block™, a liquid plastic, can be applied to the edge of your lace to keep it from fraying. I don't use it because it has a tendency to turn white. My lace doesn't fray, because I'm gentle when I'm removing it from my skin.

Get into the habit of inspecting the inside of your wig every time you remove it. Eventually, you will see small holes crop up, from your wig T-pins, or from your comb catching the lace. It's okay. Just take your clear thread and your needle, and sew that bad boy up. I do this before every application, because the lace is fragile. There will be holes. Don't sweat 'em!

There will be times when you order a wig, receive it, and try it on. Damn, it's too big... what to do? No need to send it back, just sew it up. Remember, this is basically fabric, with hair attached.

To resize your wig, make sure you have some straight sewing pins handy and follow these instructions:

1. Turn your wig inside out, with the lace on the outside, and the hair on the inside.

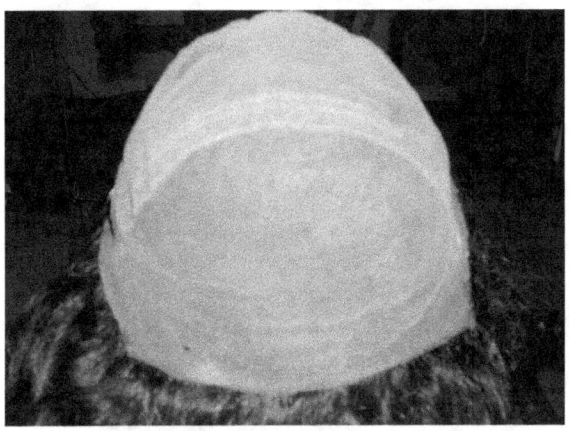

2. Make sure your hair is as flat as can be, as if you're about to install your wig.

3. Put your wig on your head. Pinch the areas of excess lace. Pinching the area, pull the wig off your head. Do not let go of the pinched area.

4. Pin off the excess lace. A good place to do this would be either behind the ears, or down the middle of the back of your head.

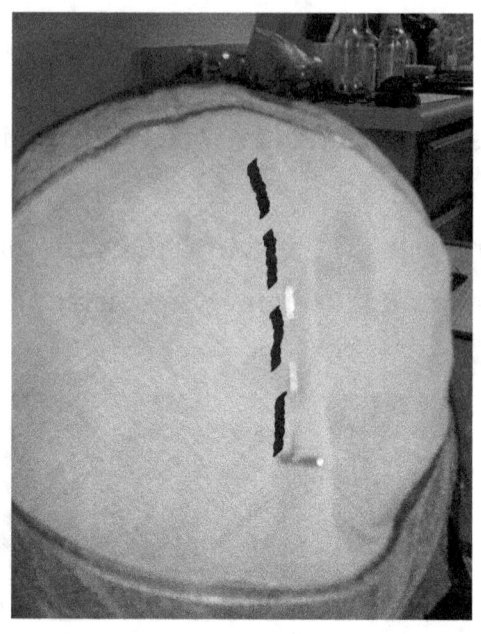

5. Sew a seam close to the pin. Sew the seam again to reinforce it.

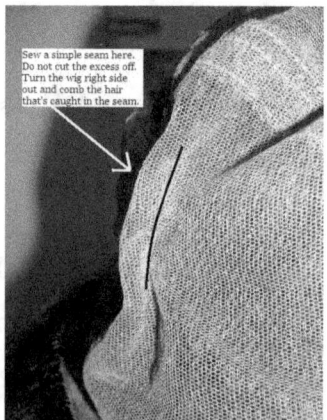

Sew a simple seam here. Do not cut the excess off. Turn the wig right side out and comb the hair that's caught in the seam.

You don't have to cut off the excess, in fact, I don't recommend cutting off the excess, because the wig will shed in that area. The excess will lay flat when you wear the wig.

Once your wigs become unwearable, you can cut them and sew them onto another wig to make a whole wig. Once I had the bleaching disaster on my virgin Malaysian loose curly, the nape area began to shed something awful. I still had the very first wig I ever bought, a virgin Malaysian wavy, in which I cut off the back to add wig clips. I ended up jacking that wig up to where I couldn't wear it anymore (cut the bangs too short). I cut off the section where the clips were, and I cut another even section across the crown of the wig, and laid it out flat on the table:

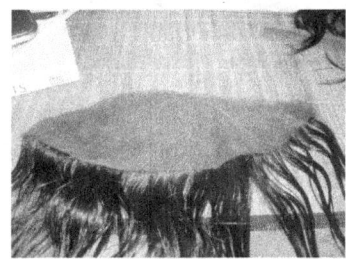 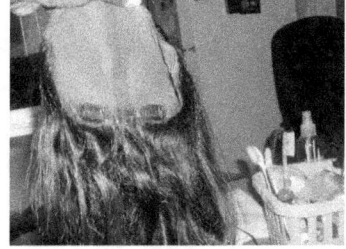

I cut the shedding section off the virgin Malaysian loose curly, and then I matched up the pieces of the two different wigs and pinned them right sides together:

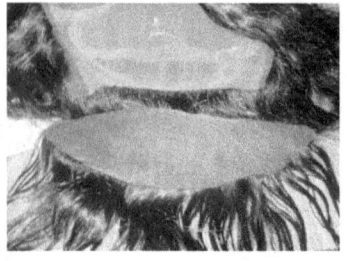 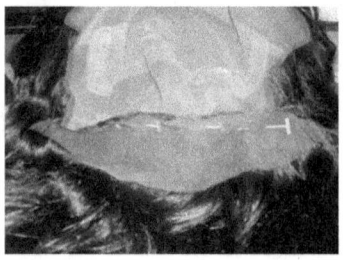

I sewed the two pieces together with clear thread first, and then I reinforced the seam with black cotton thread. After I sewed the pieces together, I trimmed the edges so they would be even:

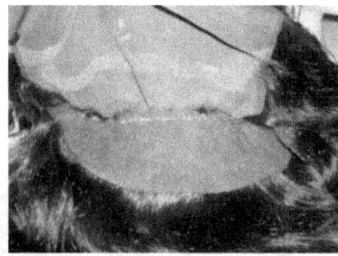 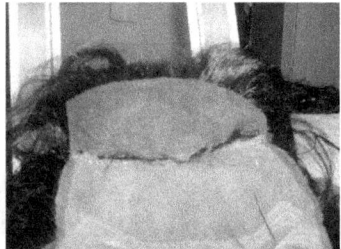

It doesn't look perfect on the inside, but on the outside, you can't tell that two different wigs have been sewn together.

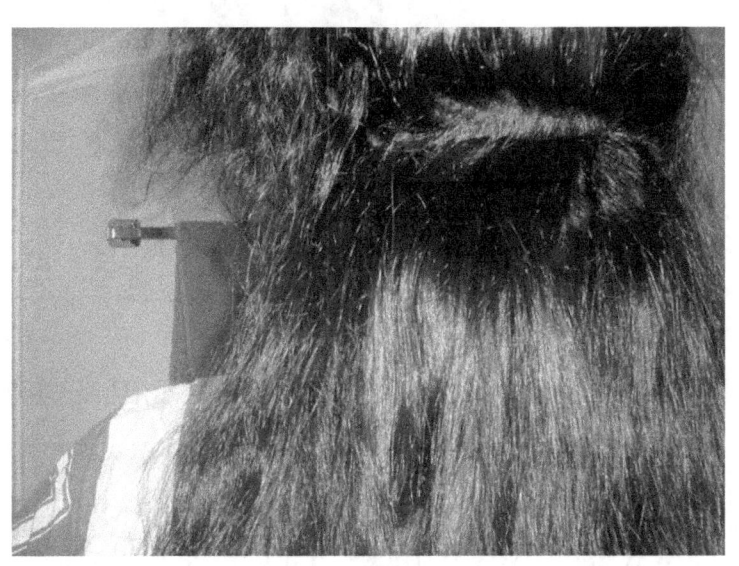

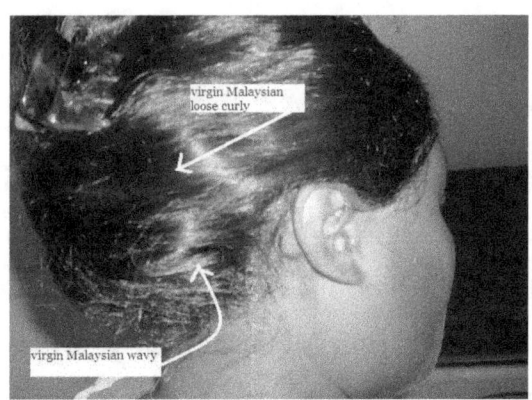

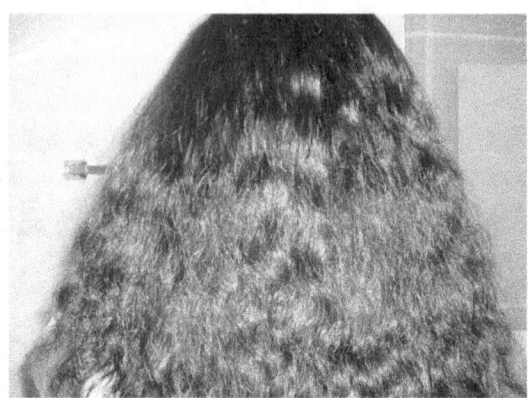

The beauty of not being afraid of the cutting the lace is if ever your wig is too small or too big, you can resize it by adding to it, or sewing a seam to make it fit correctly. You can always sew weave tracks in any area of the lace if you want fuller hair. I know several people that do this. I don't have any experience in doing this, but I know that it can be done.

Sewing Your Wig On

There are times when I want to wear my wigs, but not attach them with adhesives, tapes and clips (that hurt). It dawned on me that I could sew my wig onto my perimeter braid. My 14 inch Virgin Malaysian curly wig was ordered just for this purpose. I ordered a custom wig, because I specifically wanted a two-tone color (1B at the roots, and a 4 on the shaft of the hair), and I wanted an all lace cap with no PU strips. It didn't dawn on me to measure the front to nape and ear to ear measurement to fit that perimeter braid.

The hair came, and it was beautiful. It was closer to 16 inches. The only thing I didn't like was the hair color. It was off. That was an easy fix. I knew I was going to bleach the hair a sandy brown, with blonde highlights. The hair color portion of the experiment turned out wonderfully. Now I had to figure out how to sew it on.

I really didn't want to cut the wig; it was too beautiful. I thought about it, and I figured out that I would fold it onto itself, and then fold it back down so the edge of the lace would line up with the part behind my hairline, and in front of the braid. I prepped my hair as I would a regular application, except I left about two inches of hair out around my hairline (this would cover up the lace edge). I put my wig cap on, but I couldn't put the bandage on, which was okay, since I was showing my natural hairline. I painted the inside of the lace wig with my custom makeup blend, for my fake scalp.

Using brown weaving thread, and a weaving needle, I sewed the folded lace onto the braid, all around my head. The beehive braiding pattern is optimal for this method. I also sewed all along the fold to make sure that it wouldn't unfold.

Here's the finished look:

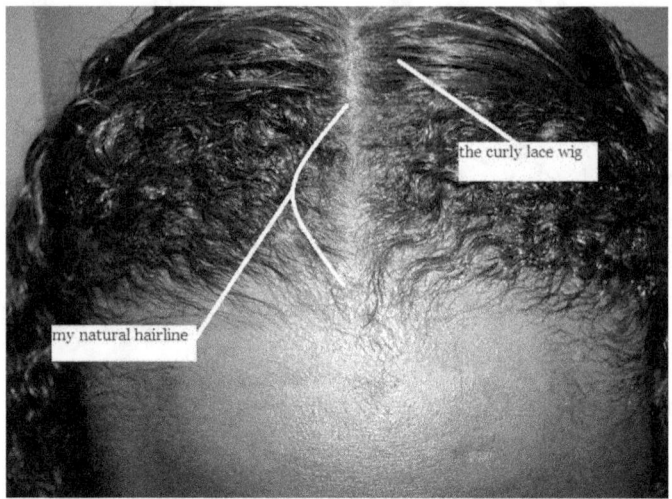

My own hair, with the 14 inch Virgin Malaysian Curly (Rex)

When I attempt this method again, I will order a wig with the correct measurements and fuller density. I think the method is a great alternative to adhesives and tape, provided you match the texture of your wig with the texture of your own hair.

Ventilating

Eventually, your wigs will "grow" bald spots. It's inevitable. Instead of throwing the wig away, consider having it re-ventilated. Ventilating is the art of hand tying hair onto the lace. This is how lace wigs are made. This seems like a logical transition for me, regarding lace wigs. Ventilating is a great skill to learn, because it can extend the life of your wigs. You can search on the internet to find people who ventilate or you can learn to do it yourself. I'm excited about this new direction, because once I learn to re-ventilate my own wigs, I will start making full lace wigs, from the first nape hair, to the last baby hair. Making my own wigs will be the ultimate in creativity, because I can design my own hairlines, and I can choose my own hair textures, densities, and colors. I'm also excited at the prospect of re-ventilating wigs and making affordable wigs for people who need them.

Part III:

Is It a Lifestyle?

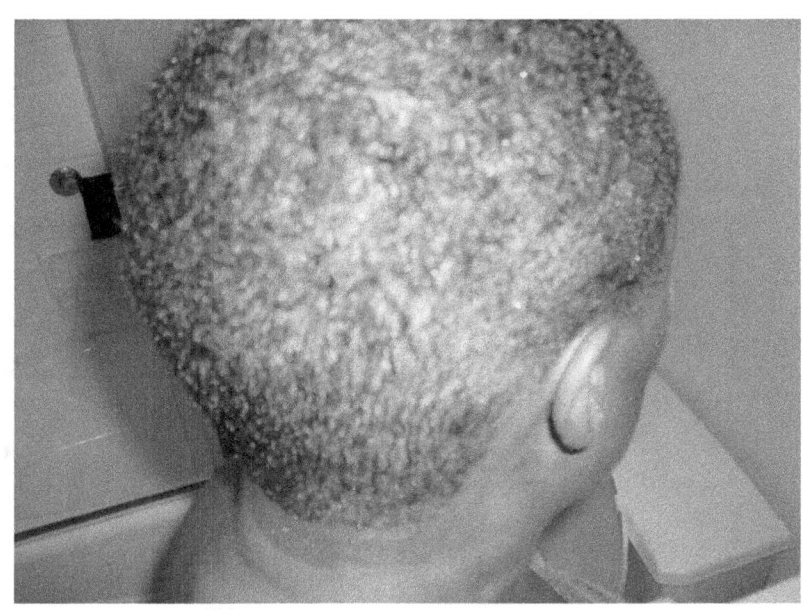

Chapter 4

My Big Chop – April 19, 2009

Ten months after starting my journey into lace wigs, I decided to chop all my hair off. The reason for such a drastic decision was that my hair was relaxed and breaking off. A couple of weeks earlier, the wrong person cut my hair, and jacked my hair UP! I had no choice but to start all over. I'd done the big chop before, so I wasn't afraid that my hair wasn't going to grow back. I didn't go through any emotional head trips when I shaved my head. I took my boyfriend's clippers and went to work. It was so liberating.

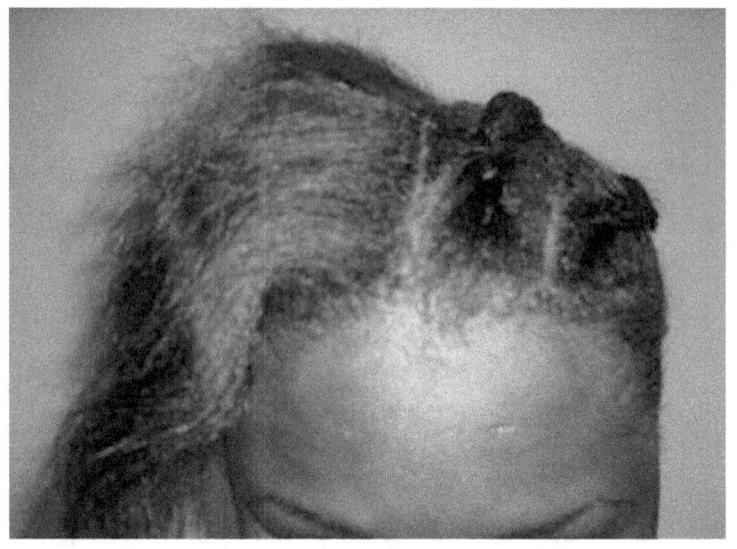

This picture was taken on April 9, 2009, right before a lace wig application, before the BC. I've always had different types of hairstyles: long, short, straight, and curly. Before the BC (as it's called), I wasn't attached to my hair. Once I chopped it all off, I found it easier to apply my lace wigs. I didn't have to wear wig caps, so I could feel air blowing through my lace, hitting my head. It felt so good. My lace on my head felt smooth, and it felt good for my boyfriend to run his hands through my (wig) hair. No braid bumps! Then my hair started to grow... and grow it did! Unless you suffer from a medical condition that prevents your hair from growing, your hair will grow, if you let it. When I hear people say "my hair won't grow", I always wonder what they're doing to their hair that causes the breakage, which makes them think their hair isn't growing. What's great about lace wigs is that your hair will grow under them, if you properly care for it. Lace wigs protect me from continuously damaging my hair. It's almost like my hair is hibernating when I'm wearing my lace wigs. I make sure my hair is moisturized under my wigs, but not to the point where my hair might mildew.

Chapter 5

Yes, I Am a Product Junkie!

Lace wigs can become an addiction. I'm including them in this section, because they're a product... THE product. You start off with your first one, in whatever texture and length. A couple of days, weeks, or months later, you buy another one, in another texture and a different length. Most all lace wig wearers I know own at least three. At one point, I had ten wigs, the majority being virgin Malaysian hair, in different textures. I eventually sold all but four of my wigs; only three are wearable. Beware of the addiction... that's all I'm saying.

Once you get your wigs situated, you begin to try and buy all kinds of products. Shampoos, conditioners (my weakness), styling aids, and styling apparatuses; the list goes on and on. As I stated earlier, I've settled on TRESemmé® Vitamin E Moisture Rich Shampoo and Conditioner for cleansing my lace wigs. I don't like to add too much styling product to the hair because product buildup can dull the shine and make the hair seem lifeless and unnatural.

I make sure I use a satin scarf to tie down my applications (and my natural hair) every night. I also sleep on a satin pillowcase.

I recently began using molecular ion steam rollers to curl my virgin Malaysian and virgin Indian straight lace wigs. The curls are long lasting, and the steam is better for the hair. Excessive direct heat can damage the hair, and cut the lifespan of your lace wig. I set the style with a light spraying of the TRESemmé® TRES TWO™ Ultra Fine Mist hair spray.

I have more products for my semi-natural hair than for my lace wigs. I am a conditioner junkie. I've learned the benefits of co-washing my hair (using conditioner to cleanse the hair, instead of shampoo). I'll wash my own hair with a clarifying shampoo after I remove the lace wig. I'll follow that up with either an extra virgin olive oil wrap (I saturate my hair with the EVOO, and cover my hair with a plastic cap, and then wrap my hair with my microfiber turban towel); or a heavy, creamy, moisturizing deep conditioner. I do this every time I remove my lace wigs. I pamper my natural hairline with a homemade natural oil mixture of grapeseed oil and jojoba oil (purchased from my local organic health food store). When I really want to treat my hairline, I put Dr. Miracle's Intensive Spot Serum around my entire hairline. I love the tingle.

Another favorite product to use on my curly hair (and my curly lace wigs) is the Denman brush. I use the Denman Medium 7. It melts my curls. It's a miracle brush. It can be found at your local beauty supply store. I use it only when the hair is wet.

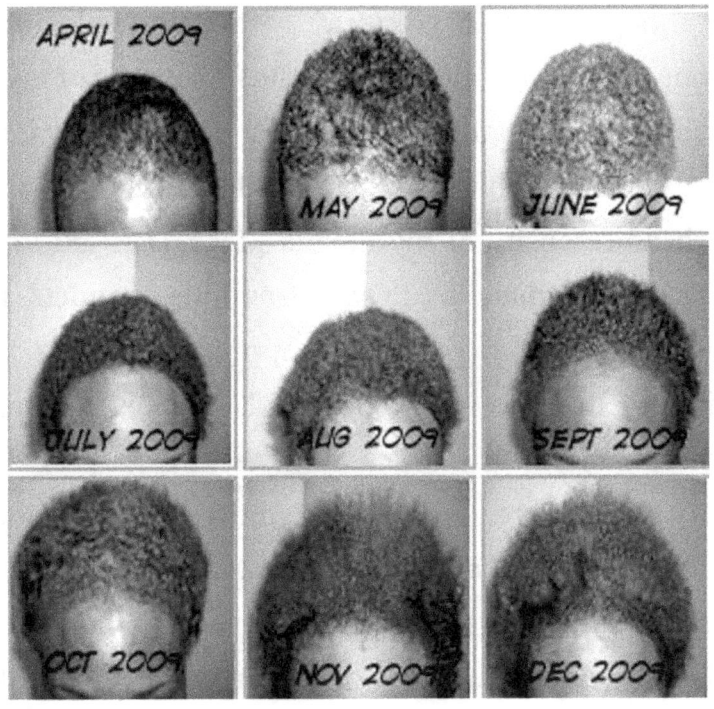

Chapter 6

My Hair's Present and Future

After I did the Big Chop, I decided that I would grow my hair back in a curly texture. My hair is a type 3c – coily, corkscrew curls. I will admit to lightly textlaxing my hair. Textlax is a method of texturizing your hair with a mild relaxer, only leaving it on for no more than five to seven minutes. Some people comb it through, some don't. The key is not to get it straight, but to release and loosen the curl pattern already imbedded in your hair. It will not add curl.

I thought I could get away with only textlaxing my hair once every four months, but the unruliness of my new growth suggests that I textlax every one to two months. One product that has made a world of difference in the growth and density of my hair is Mega-Tek Cell Equine Rebuilder. It is made by EQyss Grooming Products. I use it in between my braids before I apply my lace wig. I also use it after I remove my wig, when I want to do a protein treatment.

My hair care regimen is a bit unorthodox. I believe in the "less is more" approach. I shampoo my hair with clarifying shampoo no more than twice a month, and maybe only once a month, depending on how long I keep my braids up. I try to keep my lace wigs on my head for 8-10 days at a time, and I try to do three apps per month, keeping the same braids in the whole time. When I do take my braids down, I keep my hair out for at least a week before I re-braid and put another wig on. During that time, I put some type of conditioner in my hair everyday or every other day. When there is too much buildup, I'll co-wash my hair with a light conditioner. After rinsing the co-wash conditioner out, I'll towel dry my hair and then put either Nexxus Humectress or Aussie Moist conditioner back into my hair. I also really like Organix's Vanilla Silk conditioner too. The key is knowing when my hair needs moisture or when it needs protein. When it feels spongy, then it needs protein. When it feels dry, it needs moisture. I purchased some glycerin so I will make my own moisturizer one day. I don't like wet feeling hair, so I have to figure out a good recipe that keeps my hair soft and not wet.

I love how the lace wig journey has made me step up my game with my own hair. My hair growth goal is shoulder length textlaxed hair. I can't say that I'll ever be a completely "natural" girl; I want to be able to comfortably comb through my hair. I don't feel militant about my hair. It's mine, and I'm okay with wanting to textlax my hair. I love that when I'm not wearing a wig, I don't look like anyone else around me. My hair is coily, springy, curly, and lively. I went through a bleaching phase back in December 2009, when I covered it with demi-permanent color, so I know the light color is itching to resurface. Since the bleaching, the most processing I'll do to my natural hair is textlax and color with a demi-permanent rinse. No more straightening (that's what my straight wigs are for), and no more heat. I want to be able to pull my curly hair up into a frizzy ponytail and call it a day. Or sit at the beach and feel the ocean breeze's fingers touch my scalp. I find that wash and wear hair is the most low maintenance hair there is, and that's my hair goal. I'm getting there.

My hair, March 23, 2010 – unstretched:

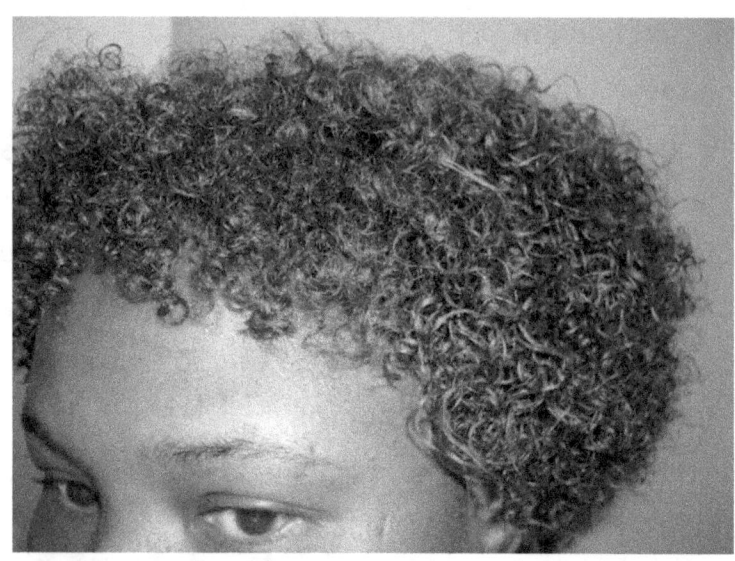

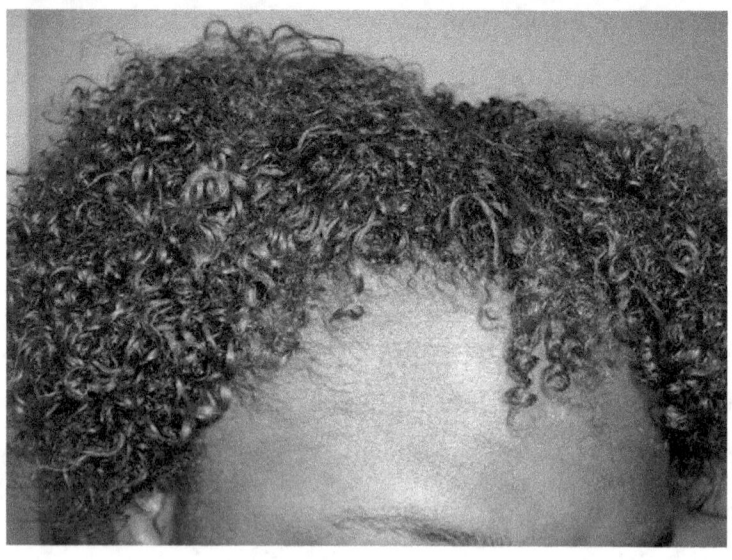

Chapter 7
Final Thoughts

Thank you for going on my hair journey with me. I hope I've answered your questions. I also hope that you use this book to guide you through your lace wig journey. Of course, once you get started, you'll outgrow this book, and that's okay. At least you have this book as a jumping off point. I didn't have a book when I started, and I sure wish I did. I'm just glad I retained all that I've learned so I could put it in a book for you. I also have a YouTube channel full of lace wig tutorials covering most of the material in this book. Continue to research, because someone's always coming up with something new regarding techniques or new products to try. The world of lace wigs is fascinating and fun.

I don't intend on wearing lace wigs everyday for the rest of my life. Once I reach my personal hair growth goal, I will wear them only when I want a change of style.

I attribute the current state of my hair to the fact that lace wigs have saved me from damaging my hair from constant manipulation and over-processing. If this is the route that you want to take with your own hair, I'm glad I could help you in your journey.

Thank you for allowing me to share with you my journey and knowledge of lace wigs and my hair.

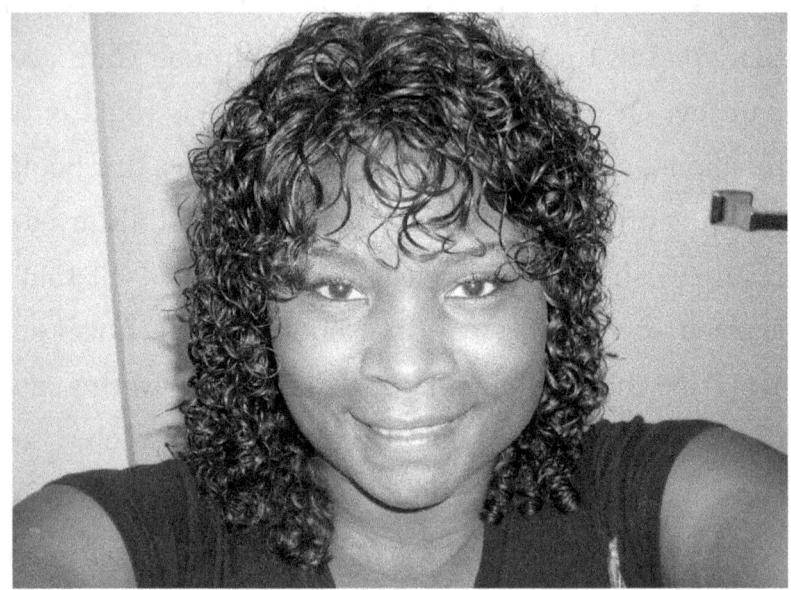

14 inch Virgin Malaysian Curly (Rex)

HOW TO MEASURE FOR A LACE WIG: Make sure you measure your head with your hair the way it will lay underneath your wig. You want your hair to lay as flat as possible. You will need a cloth measuring tape. When you measure, do not pull the tape tight, but do measure for a snug fit. We suggest you measure your head at least three (3) times for accuracy. Remember your wig will be constructed based on the measurements you submit. Also when measuring we suggest you allow ¼ of an inch beyond your hairline so when you glue your perimeter, the unit does not stick to your natural hair.

1) **Measure the circumference of your head**
   Measure all around your head. Place the tape flat against your forehead and wrap around your head. The tape should rest just above your ears and also sit on the nape of your neck.

2) **Measure front of head to nape of neck**
   Looking downward, place the tape measure approximately ¼ inch in front of your hairline at the center of your forehead, and measure back to the nape of your neck going over the crown of your head.

3) **Measure ear to ear across forehead**
   Place tape just in front of your ear at your hairline and measure across to your other ear. Bring the tape across your front hairline.

4) **Measure ear to ear over top of head**
   Place tape at your hairline directly above your ear and measure over the top of your head to the hairline above your other ear.

5) **Measure temple to temple around the back of head**
   Place the tape measure at your hairline from your temple going around the back of your head to your other temple.

6) **Measure nape of neck**
   Measure the width of your hairline across the nape of the neck.

STOCK UNIT SIZE CHART:

Cap Size	Small	Medium	Large
Circumference	21.5	22.5	23.5
Front to Nape	14	15	15.5
Ear to Ear Forehead	11.5	12	12
Ear to Ear Over Top	12	13	13.5
Temple to Temple	13.5	14.5	15.5
Nape of Neck	4.5	5	5.5

Resources

All photographs are of me, and are used with my permission.
For the color versions of these pictures, please see the Magic Hair Book photo album on my blog at http://magic-hair.blogspot.com/

My blog (http://magic-hair.blogspot.com/)

My YouTube page (http://www.youtube.com/user/Lrigyttiw#p/p)

Rex (www.junpengwigs.com)

California Lace Wigs (http://californialacewigs.com)

Hair Direct (http://www.hairdirect.com)

Black Hair Media (http://blackhairmedia.com/)

Ms Lola (http://mslola.com/)

Ms Lola's YouTube channel

(http://www.youtube.com/user/4Designers)

The Lace Wig Connection (http://thelacewigconnection.ning.com/)

Mai Lieu & the CreaClip® (http://creaclip.com/)

www.ingramcontent.com/pod-product-compliance
Lightning Source LLC
Chambersburg PA
CBHW072143280526
45788CB00002B/760